Manual of Management Counseling for the Perimenopausal and Menopausal Patient

A Clinician's Guide

Manual of Management Counseling for the Perimenopausal and Menopausal Patient

A Clinician's Guide

Mary Jane Minkin, MD
Yale University School of Medicine,
New Haven, CT

Karen L. Giblin
President and Founder of Prime Plus Inc/
Red Hot Mamas, Ridgefield, CT

The Parthenon Publishing Group
International Publishers in Medicine, Science & Technology

A CRC PRESS COMPANY
BOCA RATON   LONDON   NEW YORK   WASHINGTON, D.C.

Library of Congress Cataloging-in-Publication Data

Data available on request

British Library Cataloguing in Publication Data

Minkin, Mary Jane
 Manual of management counseling for the perimenopausal and menopausal patient: a clinician ís guide
 1. Menopause ñ Complications ñ Alternative treatment
 2. Menopause ñ Hormone therapy
 3. Perimenopause ñ Complications ñ Alternative treatment
 4. Perimenopause ñ Hormone therapy
 5. Middle aged women ñ health and hygiene
 I. Title
 II. Giblin, K aren L.
 618.1'75

ISBN 1842141813

Published in the USA by
The Parthenon Publishing Group
345 Park Avenue South, 10th Floor
New York, NY 10010, USA

Published in the UK and Eur ope by
The Parthenon Publishing Group
23ñ25 Blades Court
Deodar Road
London SW15 2NU, UK

Copyright © 2004 The P arthenon Publishing Group

Typeset by Siva Math Setters, Chennai, India.
Printed and bound in the USA

Contents

Foreword

This is a special book on women's healthcare that was written for special reasons. Mary Jane Minkin, a widely recognized specialist in menopause medicine, normally writes for her patients but this book is addressed to her colleagues. The book's tone reflects this change in purpose. Dr. Minkin is alarmed by the erosion of the intellectual approach to women's healthcare and she aims to help reverse this trend. The cause of unease among Dr. Minkin and her like-minded colleague Karen L. Giblin, a well known menopause educator, is the recent publication of several trials (the Heart and Estrogen/Progestin Replacement Study, the Estrogen Replacement and Atherosclerosis Trial and the Women's Health Initiative) that study the effects of initiating treatment with estrogen with or without progestin for reasons other than treatment of menopausal symptoms. For practical reasons the trials were performed on older and generally symptom-free menopausal women who had already been postmenopausal for 5 or more years. Many had already manifested signs of heart and blood vessel disease that the estrogen was supposed to avoid. Commencing the hormone treatment at such an advanced stage has generally turned out badly for the women who took the treatment. The reasons are complex, but they all revolve around the fact that the women in these trials had already compensated for the estrogen deficiency and had developed clinical or sub-clinical vascular disease. The response of these older women who were already afflicted with the complications of estrogen deficiency was not disease prevention; rather, the hormones aggravated the situation. This underlines the importance of starting hormone replacement therapy before cardiovascular disease takes hold, not after. Those that read this book will receive a balanced description of the way that misconceptions about these trials came about. They will understand what healthcare providers can do to respond to the questions and needs of the women who are caught in the midst of this confusion among the people that women trust to ensure their health.

Read this book. Its message has never been more important than now as more women grow older and are more in need of rational, biology-based advice and treatment. Your mothers, daughters, sisters and patients will thank you for investing the time and commitment in their health.

Frederick Naftolin, MD, DPHIL
Yale University School of Medicine
New Haven, CT
President of the North American
Menopause Society, 1998–9

1

Introduction

THE WOMEN'S HEALTH INITIATIVE

On 9 July 2002, the announcement of the termination of the estrogen/progestin (Prempro™) arm of the Women's Health Initiative (WHI) created a frenzy among menopausal women worldwide. For many, there was a belief that this was the first and only study of estrogen use to have been conducted, and that the results showed devastating effects on Prempro users. We as healthcare providers have an obligation to put this study into proper perspective for our patients, and to continue to assess new data as it becomes available in order to care for our patients properly. A brief history of estrogen use will therefore be helpful.

The approval in 1942 of Premarin® (conjugated equine estrogens) for relief of hot flashes radically altered the available options for menopausal women. On its publication in the 1960s, Dr Robert Wilson's tract entitled *Feminine Forever* was received with great enthusiasm. For women, here was the fountain of youth. However, in the 1970s, studies were reported which showed an increased risk of endometrial carcinoma in users of unopposed estrogen. This did not prove to be a major problem, as during the 1980s progestins were introduced to balance out the estrogen.

Unfortunately, progestins were associated with a multitude of problems. With the addition of cyclical progestins, women who were for the most part thrilled to have stopped having menses began to menstruate once more. The alternative of daily progestin administration seemed attractive, but this route also had its difficulties. Many women bled or at least spotted on daily medroxyprogesterone, which was the first progestin to be employed for this purpose. Nonetheless, on its introduction in 1997 Prempro (daily conjugated equine estrogens and daily medroxyprogesterone acetate) was very well received, and the market took off.

No one questioned the efficacy of combination hormone replacement therapy (HRT) for the relief of menopausal symptomatology. However, interesting data began to appear in the 1980s which suggested that women who were taking HRT had a significantly reduced risk of developing coronary artery disease (CAD). Multiple observational studies appeared which showed reductions in myocardial infarctions and in death from the latter in the range of 30–50%. This made intuitive sense, given that CAD is very rare in premenopausal women, and the incidence increases substantially post-menopausally. Epidemiologically, it was also known that women whose ovaries were surgically removed at a very young age showed a significant increase in cardiac disease.

In the 1980s we also began to see the emergence of conflicting data on the incidence of breast cancer in women on long-term estrogen. Although the majority of studies showed no significantly increased risk in women on HRT, a few papers were published that showed an increased incidence of breast cancer among long-term users.

American women have traditionally had one major fear – that of dying from breast cancer. In a typical poll taken by the Gallup organization in 1994 of women aged 45–65 years, the individuals who were surveyed estimated that 40% of women in the USA die from breast cancer. In fact, that number applies to deaths from CAD, and the actual mortality from breast cancer is around 4%.

Also appearing throughout this timeframe were multiple reports on the efficacy of HRT in the prevention of osteoporosis. As the female life expectancy increased, osteoporosis was emerging as a significant health risk. Statistics began to demonstrate that the mortality from osteoporotic fractures equaled that of breast cancer, and healthcare costs from the morbidities of bone loss escalated.

Thus the stage was set for the WHI. Wyeth Ayerst had requested the new indication from the Food and Drug Administration (FDA) for use of Premarin for the prevention of CAD. The request was denied. The FDA demanded some prospective randomized double-blinded controlled studies to prove this, so in 1993 the National Institutes of Health, with the support of Wyeth Ayerst providing the medications, began the WHI.

Two separate arms of the study were set up. In one arm, postmenopausal women with an intact uterus were randomized to receive either Prempro or placebo in a prospective double-blinded manner. In the other arm, hysterectomized women received either Premarin or placebo. In addition to the major end point of CAD, the investigators were also studying the incidence

A woman needs a physician she can confide in and trust. The doctor should be able to look at the whole picture putting all the information together to work on resolving the woman's health problems. This may require the woman inquiring about the following:

(1) Is the doctor experienced and well-trained?

(2) Does this doctor have time to listen and talk to me? Is he/she available to discuss my health problems by telephone, when needed?

(3) Does this doctor review my total health program regularly?

(4) Will this doctor allow me to build a good working partnership and share in medical decisions?

(5) When taking a medical history, does this doctor go through my entire medical history; perform a comprehensive evaluation; review symptoms and chief complaints; and inquire about my social and occupational history?

of breast cancer, stroke, venous thromboembolic disease, osteoporotic fractures and colon cancer.

Concomitantly, Wyeth Ayerst, which was certain of the efficacy of HRT for heart disease, was also sponsoring a trial of HRT for secondary prevention. Women who had documented myocardial infarctions and severe angina were administered Prempro, in an attempt to reduce the incidence of recurrent infarctions. When the results of this trial, known as HERS (Heart and Estrogen/Progestin Replacement Study), were published in 1998 they stunned most healthcare providers. Indeed, not only did Prempro not reduce the incidence of repeat coronary morbidity, but in the first year of administration the risk actually increased.

The American Heart Association and other medical groups soon responded, and HRT was pronounced an inappropriate medication for the prevention of recurrent myocardial infarctions (although if a woman was already on the drug and doing well on it, the recommendation was that it would be medically acceptable to continue its usage).

The stage was then set for 9 July 2002. A news embargo set up by the *Journal of the American Medical Association* was breached, and a story on the WHI appeared throughout the country. The study that had been started in 1993, with the aim of showing that HRT would decrease the incidence of primary heart disease, was stopped prematurely. Women who had been on the study drug Prempro for an average of 5.2 years were showing a statistically significant but only slightly increased risk of developing breast cancer. Furthermore, there was no reduction, and perhaps a slight increase, in CAD.

Although the study showed a modest decrease in hip fractures and colon cancer, the study designers had preset an automatic stop to the study if they perceived any increased risk in breast cancer. Women panicked. Phone lines to medical offices were besieged, and frustratingly for the healthcare providers who had received no advance notice of this event, physicians were bewildered about how to respond to their distraught patients.

Further anxiety was caused following the publication of the British Million Women Study in 2003 which confirmed an increased risk of breast cancer not only in estrogen/progestin users but also in estrogen-only users. This study was also the first to show a very slight increased risk of mortality from breast cancer, although this barely achieved statistical significance.

Following the announcement that the WHI study had been terminated, healthcare providers tried to reach a consensus over its interpretation. Some of them decided to tell all of their patients to come off HRT. Most healthcare providers, including the writing group for the WHI, conceded that HRT is the most effective therapy for menopausal symptomatology, and agreed to continue the usage of HRT for at least several years. The American College of Obstetricians and Gynecologists, following the WHI announcement, recommended that HRT use be limited to the relief of postmenopausal symptoms, and that its use be withdrawn as soon as possible. The North American Menopause Society (NAMS) reached a similar consensus opinion.

Many gynecologists believe that nothing really happened. Their interpretation of the initial WHI results showed nothing that we did not know previously, and they propose continued usage of HRT as they had planned prior

Women are often reluctant to ask question during their office visit with their doctor, but can be quite demanding in expecting answers. For many women, communicating their concerns does not come easy, even though they desperately look for answers from their doctors in relation to the causes, prevention and treatments of their menopausal health concerns. Often women make appointments to discuss physical symptoms, mainly for hot flashes. Unfortunately, the more difficult topics e.g., sexual issues, urogenital concerns and psychological issues fall short on the list of topics raised once they get into the doctor's office. To receive appropriate treatment, women and their doctors need to break the barriers, openly communicate and honestly address all issues which may include physical, emotional and sexual issues. Before making the appointment with the doctor, women should be armed with information and prepare the office visit in advance, with their questions and concerns written down.

When choosing a new doctor women should find out how busy that doctor really is. Appointments are sometimes hard to come by. If a woman waits more than a month to see a doctor, she may wonder whether this doctor might be too busy, God forbid, if she was seriously ill. However, many doctors specifically limit the number of new patients to allow time for their long-time patients (and in general the one who will see a new patient in less than a month is probably the less established one in practice with less experience), so a woman needs to weigh up these issues.

The first visit is important and many women feel that the allotted time should be a minimum of 30 min. The doctor who does this is usually the one who listens, and encourages patients to be active participants in their menopausal healthcare decisions. Self-esteem rises in women who become partners with their healthcare professionals. These women feel more in control, have more self-confidence and, of course, feel less frustrated. Some tips to give your patients in preparation of their visits include:

(1) When making your office visit, let the doctor's receptionist know approximately how much time you need with the doctor to discuss your concerns (although very few doctors these days will schedule more than 15 min for a return visit given insurance reimbursement issues).

(2) Have a checklist of your menopausal symptoms, concerns, and a list of all the medications you are taking, including over-the-counter herbs and vitamin supplements.

(3) Make a list of your questions and concerns that you wish to address with the doctor.

(4) If this is your first visit make sure your doctor has copies of your entire medical records prior to this visit.

(5) Bring a pen and paper to write down your doctor's comments regarding your questions and concerns. This will eliminate the need for a return visit if clarification is required about his/her responses to these concerns.

(6) Make sure you have a thorough understanding of your doctor's recommendations with regard to prescribed medications (benefits, risks and side-effects), further tests, lifestyle modifications and therapy.

to this date, accompanied by explanations to their patients. At the same meeting of NAMS that issued a statement on stopping the use of HRT, a plenary session on sexual function emphasized the importance of estrogen, and a subsequent session highlighted how important estrogen replacement therapy was for women who were surgically menopausal.

However, on 8 January 2003, almost exactly 6 months after the WHI termination announcement, the FDA pronounced that all estrogen formulations in the USA, including conjugated equine estrogens (Premarin) as well as all others, with or without progestins, should be labeled with a black box warning indicating the WHI findings. The warning would include a statement about the increased risks of breast cancer and cardiovascular disease. The statement would also recommend the use of the lowest dose of estrogen for the shortest possible amount of time for relief of vasomotor symptoms.

HOW CAN THESE DIFFERENT INTERPRETATIONS EXIST?

The increased absolute risks revealed by the WHI study are very small. According to the WHI, Prempro users experienced 38 new cases of breast cancer per 10 000 women per year, compared to 30 new cases in the control group. They also noted a similar increase in cardiovascular disease.

However, many healthcare professionals argue that breast cancer cells are present in the breast for more than 5 years prior to the discovery of the disease, and that hormonal therapy merely promotes their growth, making them detectable (and detected) earlier. They also note that in the WHI study there was no increased risk of carcinoma *in situ*, which would logically be increased if the hormones were truly carcinogenic.

Many explain the coronary data on the basis of the particular sample. The age of women enrolled in the HERS study was 67 years, whereas in the WHI the average starting age was 63 years. Although the women in the WHI did not have overt CAD, they were an obese cohort, with an average BMI of 28.5 kg/m², and 35% were hypertensive. Around 50% were current or previous smokers. Many women's health experts believe that this group most likely had some degree of plaque formation in their coronary arteries due to these risk factors. Thus they believe that the WHI is merely a confirmation of the HERS study, and that it shows no secondary protection for heart disease, but also demonstrates nothing about primary prevention.

All studies of estrogen treatement show an increased incidence of venous thromboembolic events. The range quoted in most studies is a two- to three-fold increase. The majority of these events occur during the first 6 months of use, and the WHI study was no exception. Many experts believe that the stroke data, which show a slightly increased risk in HRT users, are a consequence of the thrombogenic potential of estrogen.

WHAT DO WE TELL OUR PATIENTS?

The writing group for the WHI informed us that we should feel confident about using HRT for the relief of menopausal symptoms, and that HRT should be withdrawn when the patient is no longer experiencing significant symptoms. When interviewed, the spokespeople for the group commented that menopausal symptoms lasted for approximately 2 years, and that after this time women should be comfortable when therapy is withdrawn.

The problem is that many women who have been on HRT for a year or two for symptomatic relief are very symptomatic when therapy is withdrawn, and are still suffering from significant hot flashes, insomnia, mood swings, atrophic vaginitis and bladder symptoms. The options available include alternative therapies (both medical and non-medicinal), resumption of HRT, or allowing the patient to continue to suffer. One of the foci of this book will be how to handle the first options, since the authors firmly believe that the third choice is unacceptable.

2

Perimenopausal management

INTRODUCTION

The perimenopause consists of the years leading up to the natural cessation of menses. Symptoms commonly start in the woman's forties, can be as early as her thirties and may last for several years.

Diagnosis

No true diagnosis can be made. Menopause itself is a retrospective diagnosis. If a woman goes for one year without bleeding, in the absence of hormonal therapy, she is considered to be menopausal.

Presumptive diagnosis

If the follicle-stimulating hormone (FSH) level on day 3 of the cycle is elevated by > 12 mIU/ml, as used in infertility programs, this suggests failing ovarian function. However, this is of very limited clinical use in non-infertility settings.

Symptoms

The following symptoms are the same as those of the menopause:

(1) Hot flashes/night sweats/'crawly skin' (also known as formication);

(2) Insomnia;

(3) Irritability, mood swings/panic attacks/anxiety;

(4) Cognitive difficulties/memory lapses, fuzzy thinking;

(5) Joint aches;

My appointment is on: month ——————— day ————— year —————

Time: ———————— (a.m./p.m.) with Dr ————————————

1. How does my menstrual cycle work and interplay with my hormones?

2. What effect does aging have on my menstrual cycle?

3. What causes menopause and what factors may influence the onset of menopause?

4. How do you make a diagnosis that I am in menopause?

5. What are the symptoms that may signal that I am in menopause? Do they happen in particular sequence?

6. How do I resolve my menopausal symptoms?

7. Can you discuss hormone replacement therapy (HRT) with me – the pros, the cons and the new options?

8. Am I a candidate for HRT? Are there complementary and alternative treatments to hormone supplementation if I choose not to take HRT?

9. How do I talk to my partner, family and friends about menopause?

10. Can you offer me any other source of information and support?

Figure 1 Patient questionnaire: Questions to ask your healthcare provider about the transition into menopause

(6) Perimenstrual headaches;

(7) Palpitations, particularly premenstrually;

(8) Loss of libido;

(9) Vaginal dryness;

(10) Skin changes;

(11) Urinary tract infections, bladder control difficulty;

(12) Possibly some weight gain (some studies show a 5 to 8-pound perimenopausal gain).

Symptoms that differ from those of the menopause include bleeding difficulties such as heavy menses, prolonged menses, irregular menses (either too close together or skipped periods) and intermenstrual spotting.

Pelvic pain (distinct from atrophic symptoms) is not a classic perimenopausal symptom.

How to evaluate symptoms

There are very few objective findings on examination. Vaginal atrophy is most visible; the vagina is dry, red and friable.

A history is most helpful. If the menses are completely regular, it is less likely that the symptoms are related to the perimenopause.

Differential diagnosis

Consider the following:

(1) Stress;

(2) Depression;

(3) Caffeine usage;

(4) Excess alcohol consumption;

(5) Cocaine use;

(6) Medication side-effects:

    (a) Antihistamines (dryness);

    (b) Selective serotonin reuptake inhibitor (SSRI) antidepressants (decreased libido); and

    (c) Beta-blockers and other antihypertensives.

(7) Medical conditions, especially thyroid dysfunction. The American College of Physicians recommends screening women routinely from the age of 50 years because of the incidence of this condition (see Table 1). Depression, hair loss, weight gain and menorrhagia are classic symptoms of hypothyroidism. Palpitations and skipped menses are classic symptoms of hyperthyroidism.

Easiest way to approach therapy

Is the patient bleeding excessively or not? If she is having heavy or prolonged periods, or menses that are too close together, if she is amenable to oral contraceptives, is a non-smoker, is not significantly hypertensive, and especially if she still needs contraception, oral contraceptive pills (OCPs) are ideal therapy. However, if she is having periods at least every 20 days, is maintaining her hematocrit, is not uncomfortable and merely wants reassurance that it is safe to bleed that often, she needs no intervention.

Table 1 Medical screening procedures for menopausal patients aged 50–70 years

Screening procedure	When
Clinical breast examination	Every year
Mammogram	Every year
Breast self-examination	Monthly
Pap smear	Every year
Pelvic examination	Every year
STD (including HIV)	Whenever a woman had multiple partners, especially without condom use
Osteoporosis screening (bone mineral density test)	Every 2 years following the onset of menopause (baseline) if bone loss is demonstrated at baseline[1]
Colorectal cancer tests	Every 5–10 years
Fecal occult blood test	Every year
Cholesterol (total and HDL)	Every 5 years
Blood pressure	Every visit with doctor
Immunizations	Every 10 years for tetanus and diphtheria
Eye examination	Every year
Dental examination	Twice a year
Urine test	Every year
Skin examination	Every year
Diabetes screening	Every 3 years
Thyroid-stimulating hormone test	Every 3–5 years

[1]For a patient without risk factors a repeat of the test is only required after 5 years. STD, sexually transmitted disease; HIV, human immunodeficiency virus; HDL, high-density lipoprotein

What do you need to do before initiation of therapy?

Although endometrial pathology at this stage is not frequent in the absence of significant risk factors, most gynecologists would recommend evaluation of the endometrium.

Risk factors for endometrial hyperplasia or endometrial carcinoma include the following:

(1) Obesity;

(2) Diabetes;

(3) Hypertension;

(4) Nulliparity;

(5) Tamoxifen use.

How do you evaluate the endometrium?

(1) *Endometrial biopsy* This can be performed on most women easily in the office, particularly with the Pipelle technique. The drawback is that it only samples a small part of the endometrium, and there may be insufficient tissue. If the patient continues to bleed irregularly, even with a negative biopsy, especially in the presence of risk factors, she will require further evaluation.

(2) *Transvaginal ultrasound (TVUS)* Many practitioners can do this in the office. If not, an ultrasound facility is needed. TVUS can measure the endometrial stripe. It needs to be done at the end of the menses (timing is important). If it is thicker than 5 mm (some experts accept 6 mm), further evaluation is needed. Endometrial carcinomas have rarely been reported with an endometrium as thin as 3 mm, so if the patient continues to bleed, she will require further evaluation.

(3) *Saline hysterography* Transvaginal ultrasound is performed concomitantly with saline infusion into the uterus. Many physicians undertake this procedure in their office.

(4) *Hysteroscopy* This can be performed in the office or in a surgical center with anesthesia. It is often done with full dilatation and curettage or at least directed sampling if a polyp or other pathology is found.

How to choose oral contraceptive therapy if negative pathology is found

Dosage

Although most pharmaceutical companies will state that the lowest dose of estrogen is always best, there are very few scientific data to show that 20 μg pills have a significantly better lipid profile than 30 μg pills. The major drawback of 20 μg pills is that they are often associated with significant breakthrough bleeding, and if the patient is motivated to seek therapy for bleeding, she does not want breakthrough. Therefore if heavy and frequent menses are her chief indication, it is usually best to start with a 30 μg pill.

What progestin should be chosen?

Most will work. Choose a levonorgestrel or norgestrel pill (Nordette®, Levlen®, Lo Ovral®) if lack of libido is also an issue, as occasionally the androgenic effects of progestins may help. If bloating and PMS symptoms are a problem, drospirenone (a derivative of spironolactone) may be beneficial. Currently the only such pill is Yasmin®. If acne or facial hair are also a problem, norgestimate (Ortho-Cyclen®) may be helpful, or Yasmin.

What about tapering the dose?

After several months on a 30 µg pill with complete resolution of symptoms, it is fine to taper to a 20 µg pill.

What about women who are symptomatic with hot flashes or headaches during the placebo week?

Many perimenopausal women suffer from hot flashes or headaches around the time of their periods. If you start them on pills, these symptoms may occasionally get worse. Treatment with estrogen during the week without pills works well. Mircette®, a 20 µg desogestrel pill, comes already packaged with estradiol, 2 mg, instead of placebo pills, for five of the 'placebo' pills. If the woman is on another pill, it is easy to add either oral estradiol or patches during the week off pills. The advantage of the Climara® patch is that only one patch is needed for the 7-day pill hiatus.

When do you stop pills?

If at any time the patient wants to stop the pills, stop them. If she develops hypertension, stop them. If she is feeling well, arbitrarily the authors would stop at around the age of 51 years (average age for the onset of menopause in the USA) or at the age when her mother became fully menopausal. Wait 1 month, and then determine FSH and estradiol levels. If FSH levels are very high and the patient is very symptomatic, we would initiate HRT. If the patient is symptomatic and FSH levels are low, go back to OCPs. If the patient is well, just observe her, without any hormonal therapy. You can always initiate treatment if she starts to feel symptomatic.

Never electively stop OCPs in the summer. Ideally, try stopping them in October. This is because if the patient starts to have bad hot flashes in July, you will be unable to tell how much of this is due to the menopause as opposed to temperatures of 90°F (32°C). If she is suffering from hot flashes and it is 40°F (4°C) outside, the clinical situation is much better defined.

What if the patient is feeling great, and wants to stay on pills even if she is over 51 years of age? So long as she is a completely healthy normotensive non-smoker, we think she can remain on OCPs. We have no data to suggest that she is harming herself by doing so.

Patients without menorrhagia

What about the patient who is *not* experiencing bleeding problems, but is still having sporadic menses, and is very symptomatic (or just does not want to take OCPs)? These are actually the more difficult patients to manage, according to some experts. Some do not recommend estrogen therapy for any woman who is not fully menopausal, but obviously many women are significantly symptomatic long before final amenorrhea occurs.

Choices

Estrogen and added progestogen

Administer estrogen daily in whatever form (patch, tablet) you and your patient are comfortable with. Administer progestogen cyclically for 12 days every 2 to 3 months if the patient does not spontaneously have her own menses. Choose whatever progestin you feel is appropriate (norethindrone acetate, 2.5 mg per day for 12 days will work, as will Prometrium®, 200 mg hora somnis (natural progesterone tends to be sedating, so always start it at night and away from food intake as food increases the absorption of progesterone). Remember to remind the patient that this regime will not give her contraceptive protection, so she must continue to use contraception. Some women feel more comfortable using cyclical withdrawal every month at this point, which is fine. It is important to evaluate any abnormal bleeding.

What dose of estrogen should be used?

We usually start with estradiol, 1 mg, or esterified or conjugated estrogens, 0.625 mg, if choosing oral therapy. If the patient wants to try an even lower dosage, this is fine (0.5 mg of estradiol or 0.3 mg of esterified estrogens), but usually if she is symptomatic she will need standard dosages. If a patch is chosen, start with the 0.05 mg/day level in general (although again if the patient wishes to try the lowest dose, you can start with the 0.025 mg/day dosage). If the patient is symptomatic, increase the dose until the symptoms are under control. You can always taper the dose after the patient is comfortable (ideally for at least several months). Again, as with stopping OCPs, try not to taper or stop therapy during the summer. It is important to address individual symptoms. If the patient does not want any hormonal intervention, you can approach each symptom as you would in a fully menopausal patient.

INDIVIDUAL SYMPTOMS THAT ARE COMMON TO THE PERIMENOPAUSE AND THE MENOPAUSE

Hot flashes

Estrogen replacement therapy usually relieves hot flashes most effectively. If you start the patient on estrogen and relief does not occur, you need to look for other causes of hot flashes. Thyroid disease would be the most common cause. While checking for hyperthyroidism, also check FSH and estradiol levels. If the latter are within the premenopausal range, it is unlikely that the menopause is the cause.

Occasionally medications can cause sweating and flashes. Obtain a list of the patient's medications, including any herbal preparations that are being used. SSRIs can cause sweating. If a likely drug is found, consider tapering it off and seeing whether the symptoms respond.

In perimenopausal women, there are certain classic triggers. Hot caffeinated beverages, alcohol and hot rooms are the most common ones. Just avoiding these triggers may suffice for control.

If flashes are not severe, consider simple suggestions such as wearing layered clothing (e.g. sleeveless shirt under a sweater).

For symptoms that do not respond to simple relief measures, many patients prefer non-medical interventions, such as vitamins and herbal preparations. When evaluating data on any substances used to relieve hot flashes, you need to look at the placebo arm of the study. Any study without a placebo arm is not reliable. Almost all studies of substances for the relief of hot flashes with a placebo arm will show a reduction in either severity or number of hot flashes of around 40% with placebo. The substance studied must show a significant reduction beyond the placebo arm if it is to be considered efficacious. However, such studies do exist. Almost all studies of non-medicinal therapy are small and time limited. All of this needs to be taken into account when assessing the data.

Soy

Soy and soy derivatives are the most commonly used preparations for relief of hot flashes. Epidemiologically, the country in which women complain least of hot flashes is Japan, which has the highest dietary intake of soy in the world. Soy contains phytoestrogens called isoflavones, notably genistein and daidzein, which have estrogenic activity.

Many alternative medicine experts recommend ingesting full soy products (e.g. tofu, soy milk) for maximum benefit, as epidemiologically

16

Name _____

Date _____

Symptom	Never	Sometimes	Frequently	Always
☐ Irregular menstrual periods				
☐ Hot flashes				
☐ Night sweats				
☐ Perspiration				
☐ Vaginal dryness				
☐ Vaginal discharge				
☐ Vaginal itching/burning				
☐ Depression				
☐ Memory lapses				
☐ Fatigue				
☐ Painful intercourse				
☐ Insomnia				
☐ Heart palpitations				
☐ Joint aches/pains				
☐ Mood changes				
☐ Numbness/tingling skin				
☐ Headaches				
☐ Decreased sexual desire				
☐ Anxiety				
☐ Irritability				
☐ Dizziness				
☐ Crying spells				
☐ Frequent urination				
☐ Leaking of urine				
☐ Weight gain				

☐ Other symptoms? Please explain. _____

_____

_____

☐ List of medications you are currently taking:

Prescriptions: _____

_____

_____

Over the counter (include vitamins, supplements and herbs): ____

_____

_____

Figure 2   Patient questionnaire: menopause symptoms

mimicking eastern diets (they state that Japanese women eat whole plant products rather than extracts). However, soy is not a regular component of most western diets, so it is difficult for women in western countries to adapt. Different soy extracts have therefore been used. Most extract products list the isoflavone content. The standard recommendation is 45–60 mg of isoflavones daily for relief of symptoms. Preparations that are available in the USA include Healthy Woman, Estroven and Revival Soy.

The most controversial risk of soy is its effect on the breast. Most studies show beneficial or neutral effects on the breast. Many experts believe that soy acts as a selective estrogen receptor modulator (SERM), producing an estrogenic effect in some tissues and blocking estrogenic activity in others (namely the breast). Many point to the fact that Japanese women living in Japan have among the lowest breast cancer rates in the world, partially due to their high soy intake. (However, some believe that it is exposure to soy during the teenage years, when breast tissue differentiation actively occurs, as opposed to exposure later on in life, that is beneficial.) There are a few *in vitro* studies of breast cancer tissue exposed to soy which show increased proliferation of cancer cells. Because of this controversy, we encourage all of our breast cancer patients to consult with their oncologist before using soy to relieve their hot flashes. (Oncologists in general like to have the final say about use of all medications, including herbal preparations. This is similar to obstetricians wanting to have final clearance on any medication taken by a pregnant woman.)

The other theoretical question concerns the potential stimulation of endometrial tissue by soy, given that the latter contains phytoestrogens. Although this has not been shown, if a patient develops irregular bleeding, she should undergo endometrial sampling.

On the positive side, there are some studies which show beneficial effects of soy on the cardiovascular system. In studies primarily conducted on monkeys, data do exist on the prevention of atherogenesis.

Red clover

Red clover, available in the USA in extract form as Promensil®, contains other isoflavones, formononetin and biochanin. Although it is not available in plant form, in limited studies the extract has shown some efficacy in the relief of hot flashes. Several other studies have shown no improvement in hot flashes, so a definitive answer is not yet available.

Flaxseed

The phytoestrogens in flaxseed are lignanes. Limited data have shown a beneficial effect of these compounds in relieving hot flashes.

Black cohosh

Although it is not a phytoestrogen, in some studies black cohosh seems to show efficacy in the therapy of hot flashes. Very limited studies have been conducted in the USA, and the majority of data on cohosh come from Germany. German authors recommend its use for a 6-month period, and then recommend re-evaluation to ascertain whether it is needed any longer.

Some experts in the USA are skeptical about the benefits of cohosh, but few have noted any significant hazards. Because it is not a phytoestrogen, it steers clear of the breast cancer controversy. Nonetheless, we do recommend that our breast cancer patients discuss it with their oncologists. One study conducted at Columbia University with breast cancer patients did show a significant reduction in the severity of hot flashes in women on cohosh.

Common preparations available in the USA include Remifemin® and Estroven®.

Other vitamins

Limited as the data on soy and cohosh are, there are even fewer data on just about everything else. Many patients believe that vitamin E (at doses of 400–800 units per day) and evening primrose oil (1000 units per day) decrease hot flashes, but there is no significant literature confirming their efficacy.

Medical approaches

(1) *Bellergal S.* Available for over 30 years in the USA, Bellergal is a combination of phenobarbital and atropine. It is supposed to work as a vascular stabilizer. Side-effects include drowsiness (not a problem for bedtime dosing) and dry mouth, among other symptoms of parasympathetic activity. A typical dose is one tablet by mouth twice daily as needed.

Patients who favor this approach prefer to take the drug on an 'as needed' basis. It can be used with most other medications and herbal preparations.

(2) *Selective serotonin reuptake inhibitor/Selective norepinephrine reuptake inhibitor (SNRI) therapy* Although occasionally associated with the side-effect of sweating, most SSRIs and Effexor (venlafaxine, the main SNRI) have been studied with success with regard to the suppression of hot flashes. Standard low-dose antidepressant dosages are used. If the patient is also suffering from depressive symptoms, this may be an ideal approach to both problems.

The two main concerns we have with regard to the use of certain SSRIs in perimenopausal women are weight gain and decreased libido. The side-effect of weight gain is most commonly seen with Paxil® (paroxetine). Most perimenopausal women complain of unwanted weight gain, and if they feel that their medication is further adding to their problem, they will not want the therapy.

The other concern is decreased libido. Many perimenopausal women complain of lack of libido (see section Decreased libido on page 30), and a well known side-effect of SSRIs is potential loss of libido. If a significant loss of libido is a chief complaint as well, we would avoid SSRI therapy.

(3) *Beta-blockers* These have been used for many years to relieve vasomotor symptoms, again presumably as vascular stabilizers. If the patient also experiences headaches, beta-blockers may relieve all of their symptoms. Beta-blockers are obviously helpful as antihypertensives as well.

The downside to beta-blockers is their hypotensive effect. If your patient already has a borderline low blood pressure, these drugs may make her light-headed. Beta-blockers can also exacerbate a depressive tendency, and may lead to fatigue.

(4) *Alpha-blockers (classically clonidine)* Again these drugs have been available for many years as vasomotor stabilizers, and the same issues arise as for beta-blockers. They may have a more profound effect on the blood pressure. Alpha-blockers are now available in patch form as well as tablets.

Insomnia

We ask every patient in her forties at her annual visit what her sleeping is like. The most common answer we receive is 'Terrible – but why do you care? You are my gynecologist'. Many perimenopausal women have sleep disturbances, but do not associate these with hormonal changes.

The classic perimenopausal sleep pattern is that a woman will fall asleep readily and early, as she is exhausted. She then wakes up at 1 or 2 a.m., cannot fall asleep again for 1 or 2 h, finally falls asleep at 4 a.m., and then wakes up to go to work at 6 a.m., after which she is fatigued all day. This pattern can normally be readily differentiated from a depressive insomnia, which is usually associated with difficulty falling asleep and with early-morning wakening.

Sometimes this sleep disruption will be accompanied by hot flashes, while at other times the woman will just awaken spontaneously. Some sleep research has shown that even in women who do not report insomnia, the quality of menopausal sleep is poorer.

Again HRT is usually successful. For the patient who does not want HRT, there are other options. One variant of HRT can be helpful. For decades, natural progesterone has been known to cause somnolence (many years ago anesthesiologists used it as an adjunct for sedating their patients). Therefore if a woman is willing to take natural progesterone before sleep, this may help. If the woman wants a commercially available natural progesterone, Prometrium is available with a prescription. Many women prefer a compounding pharmacy version, in a cream or lozenge form, which is also fine. However, there is no guarantee about the stability and content of progesterone in compounded form. If there is no improvement in sleep after taking compounded progesterone, an assessment may be difficult.

Lifestyle changes

The more active a woman is during the day, the better she will sleep at night. However, you should encourage her to exercise early in the day (or at least before dinner), because evening exercise may make it more difficult for her to fall asleep.

Herbal alternatives

(1) *Soy (see section on hot flashes)*   The data for relief of insomnia by soy are weaker than the hot flash data. However, it is still worth finding out whether soy will help. Use the same standard amounts that are recommended for hot flashes. Similar statements would apply to other isoflavones.

(2) *Cohosh*   As with soy, cohosh seems to have better efficacy for relief of hot flashes than for sleep improvement, but again, because it is a reasonably safe option, it is quite sensible to try it. Use the same dosages as recommended for hot flashes.

(3) *Melatonin*   Although it is a relatively safe alternative approach, the sleep response to melatonin is very variable. It is quite reasonable to try this approach (the standard dosage is 1 to 3 mg), but do not expect astounding results.

(4) *Other traditional herbal approaches (non-specifically for menopause)*   Many herbalists will recommend valerian, chamomile and motherwort as options. The data on these approaches are mixed, but these herbs are unlikely to produce toxicity in your patients.

Medical approaches

(1) *Bellergal S.*   Bellergal is primarily used as a medication for hot flashes. However, as one of its main side-effects is sedation, at night it may provide a better night's sleep as well.

(2) *Hypnotics*   Any sleeping medication will help to relieve perimenopausal insomnia. The major drawbacks are of course habituation to the drug and side-effects, such as drowsiness the next day. If a woman has had a series of difficult nights, it may be helpful to prescribe hypnotics for her for short-term periodic usage, with an explanation of the drawbacks of therapy.

A relative newcomer to the hypnotic market is zaleplon (Sonata®). The advantage of this medication over some others is its relatively short half-life. A woman can take it if she is awake at 1 a.m., and be able to awaken again at 6 a.m.

One caution should be given about over-the-counter sleep aids. Many patients take antihistamines to help them to sleep. One of the most commonly used medications is Tylenol PM®, which consists of Benadryl plus Tylenol. Antihistamines can lead to mucous membrane dryness, and menopausal women often complain of dryness as a separate symptom, so in this case relieving one symptom may exacerbate another.

Alcohol use

Perimenopausal women are at high risk of becoming dependent on alcohol, and one of the problems that can drive them that way is sleep disruption. Question your patient about her alcohol use, if you have any prompts which lead you in that direction, and offer to help her to solve her sleep problem without developing a reliance on alcohol.

Irritability and mood swings

For many years the American Psychiatric Association listed as an official diagnosis 'involutional melancholia', or depressive symptoms associated with the menopause. They withdrew this diagnosis several years ago. However, recent research has shown that some perimenopausal women fail to respond to standard antidepressant medication unless they have been repleted with estrogen, so psychiatrists are once again beginning to think of some link between depressive symptoms and the menopause. Even among those psychiatrists who believe that depression will not arise *de novo* during the menopause, most agree that women with a history of depression may well experience a recurrence at menopause.

A careful recording of symptoms is required in these women. Are they exhausted due to sleep deprivation? If they are totally sleep deprived, getting sleep is crucial, and this may cure their mood swings.

Is the woman still experiencing some menstrual activity, and are her symptoms exacerbated premenstrually? Charting here is crucial, because she may have significant premenstrual syndrome (PMS) or premenstrual dysphoric disorder (PMDD). For these women, therapy with SSRIs has been shown to be most effective, and can be used in an intermittent dosage schedule if the patient so wishes. Both fluoxetine (Prozac® or Sarafem®) and sertraline (Zoloft®) have been shown to be effective, both as a daily regime and intermittently.

Of course, women in their mid- to late forties, and throughout their fifties are subject to significant external stresses. It is crucial to know exactly what is going on in your patient's life. She may have returned to the workforce after her children have gone off to school or work, or her partner may be dealing with a lay-off from work. Her children may be going off to school, or coming back, or asking her to provide daycare for their offspring, or she may be dealing with aging parents and in-laws. She may be developing other medical illnesses. All of these can be stress factors, and in order to help her to sort out what is going on, you need to know what is happening. If there are significant stress factors which are interfering with her daily activity, see if you can put her in touch with a counselor. Most health maintenance organizations (HMOs) have counselors (e.g. social workers, psychologists) affiliated with them who can help women to sort out these difficulties. Menopausal support groups, such as Red Hot Mamas, can also be helpful.

Regular exercise is always helpful for dealing with stress. If she engages in aerobic activity during the day, the woman will sleep better at night.

Regular aerobic activity (aiming at 30–45 min of vigorous activity four or five times per week) will help her to deal with stress more effectively. If ailing parents or in-laws are the cause of her stress, exercising will help her to realize that the ills of these older people will be less likely to befall her.

Other lifestyle changes can also be helpful. Many women find that meditation can help them. So can joining a support group to help to deal with some of the stresses, and the realization that other women are dealing with very similar issues.

Herbal management

St John's wort has been used extensively in Europe as an antidepressant. There are reasonable data to demonstrate its efficacy. Its mechanism of action is not entirely clear, and it should not be used by individuals who are on monoamine oxidase (MAO) inhibitors. The major problem in the USA is that most people use brands with significantly varying doses of active ingredient. If your patient would like to try St John's wort, encourage her to try a well-recognized brand that contains reliable amounts of the drug. This drug should also not be used in conjunction with SSRIs.

Valerian root has been used for many years as an anti-anxiety agent. However, it also has the problem of very variable doses in preparations available in the USA. Unlike the herbal products discussed above, a number of significant side-effects, including congestive heart-failure, have been demonstrated, so it is not recommended as a sedative in general for long-term therapy.

Vitex has been used in Germany to 'regulate hormonal levels', and is recommended for the treatment of menstrual irregularities and menopausal symptoms. It is important to remember though that one of the other common names for vitex is chasteberry, and this drug has been reported to lower libido levels. So if decreased libido is another major complaint of the patient, one would want to avoid vitex.

Medical management

HRT will usually help if the mood swings are clearly related to insomnia. It may also help in certain other situations, and this is one of the scenarios in which we will often advocate that a patient tries hormonal intervention for a month or two to see whether her symptoms abate. Even if she chooses to stop HRT after 2 months, and her symptoms were solved by this therapy, she now knows the cause of the emotional symptoms.

(1) *Antidepressant therapy* Formerly, if you felt that a patient was depressed enough to require antidepressant therapy, you would automatically refer them to a psychiatrist. Depending on your patient's insurance coverage, you may not now have that luxury. Even if she has mental health coverage, it may only be for a counselor who cannot prescribe medication. Therefore it is helpful for all medical personnel who can prescribe medications and who treat perimenopausal and menopausal women to know the basics of antidepressant and anxiolytic medications.

Fortunately, SSRIs, which are the current mainstay of treatment, are quite safe compared with the formerly used tricyclic antidepressants. Overdoses are unusual, and side-effects can be annoying but are seldom life-threatening. Initiate therapy at a low dose, and if one drug does not work, taper the patient off and try another. Remind the woman not to expect significant results for 2 to 4 weeks (PMDD responds much more quickly than true depression). Side-effects may include fatigue, weight gain (most commonly seen with paroxetine (Paxil), but can also be observed with any SSRI), constipation and loss of libido.

Practitioners usually find several SSRIs with which they are comfortable. Fluoxetine (Prozac) was the original SSRI, and has now also been approved for use to treat PMDD. It has a relatively long half-life, and is available in once-a-week as well as daily dosing.

Sertraline (Zoloft) and paroxetine (Paxil) have been used as antianxiety agents as well as antidepressants. Citalopram (Celexa®) has been used in Europe prior to its use in the USA. Escitalopram (Lexapro®) is a derivative of Celexa.

Venlafaxine (Effexor) has the activities of both an SNRI and an SSRI. Widely used to treat hot flashes in women who cannot or do not wish to take HRT, it also has good antidepressant properties.

For women who experience side-effects with SSRIs, a drug such as bupropion (Wellbutrin™) may prove helpful. For a woman who has a decreased libido to begin with, an SSRI may make her situation worse, and Wellbutrin would be a better drug. Wellbutrin is also used for smoking cessation, so if your patient is a smoker, you may help her to quit as well. If a woman is happy with her SSRI in general but has problems with reduced libido as a side-effect, the addition of Wellbutrin to her regime may prove helpful.

(2) *Antianxiety medications* As mentioned above, certain SSRIs have the added benefit of antianxiety effects. For the woman who has only occasional problems with anxiety, occasional use of a benzodiazepine

can help. Drugs such as alprazolam (Xanax®) or lorazepam (Ativan®) are very inexpensive and effective acute antianxiety drugs. The standard dosage for both would be one tablet (0.5 mg) every 6 h as needed. However, the downside of any benzodiazepine is the side-effect of depression and fatigue. These medications can also be habituating, so if the woman finds that she needs to take these medications round the clock, she would probably be better off with sertraline or paroxetine. Occasionally a woman may feel that she does better on regular benzodiazepines. We feel that these patients are better managed by a psychiatrist because of the potential for habituation.

Some psychiatrists recommend buspirone (Buspar®) for anxiety. In general our patients have not responded well to this drug. It has minimal side-effects, but patients do not generally report substantial relief of anxiety.

Cognitive difficulties

This is an extremely controversial area of perimenopause and menopause management. Do estrogens and androgens have central nervous system effects? Certainly there are well-documented hormone receptors throughout the brain. Women who are going through the menopause regularly complain of difficulty with thinking and memory loss.

Certain classical experiments have been conducted on the effects of estrogen on memory, which showed that estrogen and testosterone improve memory function in women after bilateral oophorectomy. However, many researchers claim that the cognitive declines are related more to aging than to loss of hormones.

Many practitioners prescribe HRT for loss of cognitive functions. Unfortunately, there is very little else to offer for therapy. If the woman has severe memory loss or cognitive dysfunction, referral to a neurologist or psychologist for psychometric testing is very appropriate. Alzheimer's disease may be diagnosed in women in their fifties. For true dementia, medications such as donepezil (Aricept®) and rivastigmine (Exelon®) have been shown to slow progression of the disease, making the diagnosis relevant.

However, the picture is less clear for the woman with moderate cognitive difficulties. The data on *Ginkgo biloba* are very sketchy. Traditional medicine has little to offer here either. If you do start your patient on hormonal therapy and she responds, we would suggest that you maintain it for at least a few months, and then taper the dose down slowly and see how the patient responds.

Of course, lifestyle approaches can be helpful here, as in most other areas. Regular physical exercise can improve concentration, and mental exercises (to improve memory) can be helpful. Remember that one of the complaints about many studies of Alzheimer's disease and estrogen is that these investigations are confounded by the fact that many estrogen users are also more mentally active (e.g. going to book or chess clubs, which in and of themselves can improve thinking).

Joint aches

Joint aches and arthritic-type pains are extremely common in women in their late forties and their fifties. This is another group of symptoms that is difficult to ascribe to menopause as opposed to mere age-related changes. The classic Australian study in which women were monitored as they aged, comparing e.g. a 50-year-old premenopausal woman with a 50-year-old post-menopausal woman, would suggest that somatic changes may be more related to the aging process.

The role of HRT here is also rather unclear. Traditionally, as rheumatoid diseases such as lupus or rheumatoid arthritis are more common in women, many authorities state that estrogen can exacerbate these types of diseases. However, in more common osteoarthritis, some believe that estrogen can ameliorate symptoms by moistening synovial membranes, just as it lubricates other mucous membranes, and that it can help to relieve joint pains. This is another area in which empirical therapy may be warranted, depending on how debilitating the patient's symptoms are.

Arthritic complaints cause many women to seek complementary and alternative approaches. Chiropractic therapy can be very helpful here. Of course, good allopathic physical therapy is an excellent approach as well. A prescribed set of exercises performed on a regular basis can alleviate a significant number of these aches and pains. You must also emphasize weight loss to the overweight patient with joint aches, as the less pressure the body exerts on a joint, the less it will hurt.

Many women will complain that they ache too much to exercise. For these patients, swimming or aquatic aerobics are ideal. Many Young Men's Christian Associations (YMCAs) have organized water aerobics classes, and the programs will usually ease joint pain and help the patient to lose weight.

For the patient who desires alternative medication, glucosamine has been shown to work in some prospective randomized trials. With doses ranging from 500 to 750 mg twice daily, many patients will show a clinical response.

Many of your patients will be familiar with this approach, as their dogs have already been taking it (veterinarians have recommended glucosamine for animal arthritic complaints for years).

For the patient who needs medication for symptom relief, non-steroidal anti-inflammatory drugs (NSAIDs) have been the mainstay of therapy for many years. Ibuprofen and naproxen lead the over-the-counter therapies. During the past 3 years, the COX-2 inhibitors have made inroads in the arthritic market. Theoretically, it was felt that these drugs, namely cele-coxib (Celebrex®), rofecoxib (Vioxx®) and valdecoxib (Bextra®), were somewhat safer than the standard NSAIDs, which had both COX-1 and COX-2 activity. However, current studies have documented that a significant gastrointestinal bleeding risk exists with even selective COX-2 inhibitors. Of course, all non-steroidal drugs have been potentially associated with renal disease if used on a chronic basis. For these reasons, we try to avoid long-term round-the-clock NSAIDs. Referral to a rheumatologist would certainly be indicated for patients with such debilitating complaints.

Perimenstrual headaches

Many women with chronic migraines have long since figured out that their headaches have a significant menstrual association. Although not all migraines are related to the menstrual cycle, for many women the 2 days before their period and the first day or two of their menstrual flow can lead to a significant headache. These patterns may become exacerbated as these women become menopausal, and some women who were never previously migraine sufferers develop this pattern as they reach the perimenopause.

Our mentor Dr Philip Sarrel and his neurology colleagues at Yale, notably Dr Lawrence Brass, among others, have spent some considerable time studying these women. Many years ago Dr Sarrel measured estrogen levels in women who complained of these perimenstrual headaches. He also attached these women to vascular monitors, and found that many of them had very low blood estradiol levels as well as decreased cerebral flow. He then administered sublingual estradiol to these women, which is the quickest non-parenteral means of administration. He found that as their estrogen levels increased, their cerebral blood flow increased and their headaches resolved.

Migraine sufferers should be encouraged to keep a diary of their attacks. If a clear pattern becomes apparent, these women can be given estrogen for

2 or 3 days premenstrually, and through the first day or two of their periods, when they seem to experience symptoms. You can administer estradiol orally, 1 mg once or twice a day, or these women can place an estrogen patch around the time when they would become symptomatic, and remove it when they would no longer need it for symptomatic relief. A 0.05 mg/day patch is usually sufficient for therapy.

If a woman has an acute attack, sublingual administration will work most quickly. If you do use a sublingual dose of 1 mg, ideally ask your patient to swallow another 1 mg tablet when she is able to do so. If you do not administer an oral dose, the sublingual dose tends to wear off quickly, and she may become symptomatic shortly afterwards. Obviously, for sublingual administration you cannot use any form of coated estrogen tablet, as it will not be absorbed. A good non-coated estrogen to use may be Estrace®.

These types of headaches are also commonly seen in oral contraceptive users (see the above section on OCP use for control of menorrhagia). The same brief estrogen replacement regime will work for many of these women. This is why you must ask a patient who complains of headaches on OCPs when she gets her headaches. The patient who develops headaches during the pill weeks may do better off the pill, and should stop pill usage in order to evaluate this. However, for the patient who develops symptoms during the week off the pill (or during the placebo week), stopping pill use may not help at all, but perimenstrual estrogen will often work.

Of course, if estrogen therapy does not stop the attacks completely, other methods of symptomatic relief can be tried. The patient can use tryptan therapy, such as sumatriptan (Imitrex®) and its derivatives. Women with a history of chest pains or cardiac disease should not use tryptans. For many women, butalbital (in Fiorinal® or Fioricet®) will work well as back-up therapy. Any patient with a new onset of headaches which are not clearly completely relieved by estrogen therapy should be evaluated neurologically. Any one severe headache mandates neurological evaluation.

One of the many uses of the drug *Botulinum* toxin (Botox®) has been for migraine therapy. It is used for muscular blockade, and may have a relaxing effect that contributes to headache relief. This therapy is currently primarily prescribed by neurologists.

Palpitations

For some women, the catecholamine release that leads to hot flashes can also lead to palpitations, and some women will develop palpitations without any hot flashes at all. Classically, for the perimenopausal woman, these palpitations will usually occur immediately before her periods, in general at the nadir of her cyclical estrogen production.

As women can develop heart disease as they approach menopause, any woman with palpitations should undergo a cardiac evaluation. A set of thyroid function tests will be useful, as hyperthyroidism can cause palpitations. If your patient has not had a recent lipid profile, it would be useful to repeat one of these, too, so that cardiologists can quickly devise their work-up when they see the patient, armed with the results of these blood tests.

In the absence of cardiac problems, a trial of estrogen can be useful here. Some women with a clear-cut perimenstrual pattern can be treated just like migraineurs, using low-dose oral or patch estradiol. Some women will do better with estrogen augmentation all month. You can try 1 mg a day of estradiol or a 0.05 mg/day patch on an ongoing basis for 1 or 2 months, and ask the patient to record her symptoms in a diary.

Alternatively, you can use low-dose beta-blockers in this situation. Many medical practitioners who are anxious about public speaking have been known to take 10 or 20 mg of propranolol or 25 or 50 mg of atenolol before their talks. A similar low dose of beta-blockers, taken once or twice a day, can help the patient with palpitations. Of course, you can use estrogen and beta-blockers together, if one of these drugs alone does not provide complete relief.

Alternative approaches are not notoriously reliable for this complaint. One can of course use soy in this situation, but the results obtained have been mixed. Biofeedback therapy can be helpful here.

Decreased libido

When the maker of a new device to help improve libido came to speak with us about this problem, he asked us how many patients consulted us about this problem on a daily basis. We thought about his question and answered 'Probably about five a day, on average'. He was astounded by our answer – but we think that we were perhaps underestimating. Given that most studies of women show an incidence of female sexual dysfunction of around 40%, the number is hardly surprising, and the problem is quite common in peri- and postmenopausal women.

No one knows exactly what hormones are responsible for sexual desire. Some believe that the latter is truly all cerebrally driven without any sex-hormone involvement, but most ascribe some role to estrogen, testosterone and dehydroepiandrosterone (DHEA).

The first question you must ask of the patient who presents with this complaint is 'Does it hurt to have sex?'. If the woman is suffering from vaginal atrophy, you must first help her to relieve this problem (see next section). As we say to our patients, 'Only a crazy person would want to do something that is painful'.

Also when asking your initial questions you should find out whether the patient and her partner are bothered by this decrease in libido. For many women, their partners are equally disinterested in intercourse. A decrease in libido by itself is not a problem if it does not bother the woman or her partner. It is only an issue if the levels of sexual interest are unequal. For many women in the pre-Viagra era, sexual (dys)function was not a problem. It was only when their partners became more sexually interested that their lack of libido was unmasked.

However, the more common complaint is the following: 'I am totally comfortable with intercourse, and as a matter of fact, once we get going I have a good time. It's just I have no interest in starting the process'. Obviously, relationship issues need to be explored, and intercurrent stress factors that can interfere with a relationship need to be discussed. However, if the patient's life is otherwise good, medical aspects need to be investigated.

Some medical illnesses and their therapies can decrease libido. If the patient has galactorrhea, or is taking any psychotropic drug, check her prolactin level (indeed, decreased libido is one of the hallmarks of diagnosis of a pituitary adenoma in men). If there are any other symptoms that raise the suspicion of thyroid disease, perform a set of thyroid function tests and check the thyroid-stimulating hormone (TSH) level. If the patient is hypertensive, find out which drugs she is taking. Classically, alpha- and beta-blockers can blunt her responsiveness. A woman with significant diabetes may have sexual dysfunction, and tighter control of her diabetes might help.

Among the largest groups of medications that decrease libido are SSRIs. Although different companies assert that their particular brand has less effect on libido, any SSRI can have these effects. Of course, depression itself can cause loss of libido, and for many women the decreased libido antedated their SSRI usage.

If loss of libido is a problem with SSRI usage, you can taper the patient off the drug and evaluate her libido and depression off the medication. If she is still depressed but her libido is increased, you can try a different SSRI to see if she reacts in the same way to the drug. Another option is to try the

31

non-SSRI antidepressant bupropion (Wellbutrin), which does not depress libido. Yet another option is to maintain the patient on the SSRI if she is feeling well with it for her depression, and *add* bupropion to it, which some psychiatrists feel does help with libido.

There have been a few studies of the use of sildenafil (Viagra®) in women who are taking SSRIs, for improvement of both libido and orgasmic response. The results have been mixed. Again, as this drug has not been approved for use in women, this would be an 'off-label' use, but after discussion with your patient you could consider some empiric therapy.

However, in the absence of medical or psychological problems, HRT should be discussed. Many authors advocate checking hormone levels, particularly of testosterone (total and percentage free) and DHEA and DHEA-S (dehydroepiandrosterone sulfate). Many women shudder at the mention of testosterone in this context. We explain to them that there are very few hormones in nature which are sex-exclusive, and we point out to them that a 70-year-old 'postmenopausal' man has much higher levels of estrogen than a comparable 70-year-old woman. You can also explain that there have been studies in the literature endorsing replacement of estrogen, testosterone and DHEA to improve libido.

Most women will then ask for a detailed account of the side-effects of testosterone therapy. The most common concern they express is anxiety that they may wake up looking like Osama Bin Laden. You need to reassure them that if they do develop any facial hair, this process will usually be quite gradual. You should also reassure them that the doses we use for testosterone supplementation are much lower than the typical male replacement doses. In addition, you should tell them that they may notice a deepening of the voice, or perhaps subtle aggressive changes (which some patients actually view very positively). Again, with low-dose therapy these side-effects are rare.

Many women are reluctant to initiate estrogen therapy, whereas they will agree to try testosterone. In the perimenopausal patient who still has significant amounts of estrogen, this may be less of an issue than in the fully menopausal woman who has a very low estrogen level. There are several notable experts who believe that a woman must have some estrogen available for sexual responsiveness, and that testosterone therapy alone will not work. However, it is still reasonable to initiate testosterone replacement for the woman with low testosterone levels. Many will initiate therapy empirically.

Most experts who deal with libido issues will advocate use of the therapy for at least a 3-month trial period (assuming that there are no adverse reactions in the interim), pointing out that the change in responsiveness will take up to

Personal details

Name _____

Address _____

Phone _____

Date of birth _____

Height _____

Weight _____

Blood type _____

Medical conditions _____

Current medications _____

Past medications _____

Allergies _____

Menstrual history (onset or any recent changes) _____

Reproductive health (number of pregnancies, birth,
  miscarriages, abortions) _____

Birth-control history (present/past methods) _____

Hormone replacement therapy (present/past methods) _____

Surgical procedures _____

Test results

☐ Blood pressure _____

☐ Pap smear _____

☐ Breast examination _____

☐ Mammography _____

☐ Complete blood count _____

☐ Hemoglobin _____

☐ Hematocrit _____

☐ Ferritin _____

☐ Cholesterol level _____

☐ High-density lipoprotein level _____

☐ Low-density lipoprotein level _____

☐ Urine test for calcium-to-creatinine ratio _____

☐ Vaginal pH/maturation index _____

☐ Follicle-stimulating hormone profile _____

☐ Thyroid profile _____

☐ Blood glucose level _____

☐ Abnormalities in blood chemistry _____

☐ Stool test (occult blood) _____

☐ Bone density measurement _____

☐ Hearing and vision check-up _____

☐ Cardiovascular testing _____

☐ Sigmoidoscopy _____

Figure 3 Profile of a patient's medical conditions and history

3 months to notice. This is why 'as-required' use of testosterone (which many patients would prefer to use) rarely works (in more than a placebo response).

Unfortunately, testosterone therapy is still not that simple to initiate for women. For the woman who is already taking estrogen, or who wishes to initiate estrogen therapy as well, there is a drug called Estratest®. This contains 1.25 mg of esterified estrogens and 2.5 mg of methyl testosterone (Estratest HS, or half-strength, contains half the amount of both medications). Methyl testosterone has been associated with hepatic dysfunction, but the latter is rare at these low doses.

A testosterone patch for female use has been tested in research protocols, and is supposed to be launched on American markets shortly, but at the time of writing it is still unavailable. There are testosterone patches available for men, but obviously these have levels that are too high for use in women.

Many practitioners have for years relied on various injectable and transdermal compounded testosterone gels and creams. Monthly injections of testosterone have been used in many areas of the southern USA, but are rarely used outside these areas. Most gynecologists rely on a good compounding pharmacy. It is a good idea to get to know the best compounding pharmacies in your area, because most of the big-chain pharmacies will not synthesize the medication you would like to prescribe. There are several national compounding pharmacies if you cannot find a good local pharmacy. For many years, the Women's International Pharmacy (1-800-279-5708) in Madison, WI, has compounded many hormonal preparations and will send them to your patients in the mail.

One of the problems your patients may face with compounded medications is that their HMOs will not pay for them. This is something that your patient will need to check with her insurance company.

The standard testosterone preparation is in general prepared at a concentration of 1–2%, in a petrolatum base. Again, however, discuss with your local compounding pharmacist what products he or she can prepare for you. Many gynecologists recommend applying the dose to the lower abdominal wall. However, as many patients have told us that vulvar application seems to enhance local responsiveness, we ask them to try vulvar application daily. Most gynecologists feel comfortable with this, as we have used topical testosterone applied to the vulva to treat lichen sclerosis et atrophicus (LS and A) for years. Again, 'as-required' application does not usually work, so they should try daily applications.

Because this is not methyltestosterone, you do not have the concern with transdermals of liver function abnormalities. One concern that some practitioners do have is lipid abnormalities, just because androgens are being prescribed. As these are peri- and postmenopausal women, they should be having regular lipid profiles in any case. If significant exacerbation of their lipids was found, you might consider stopping their androgens, but in general the small doses used for women seldom cause significant abnormalities.

A commercially available preparation called AndroGel® (testosterone, 1%) has been introduced recently for male hypogonadism. It comes in a packet, with the recommendation that the contents be applied to the abdomen. The directions for male usage are one packet to be applied daily. Some practitioners have started to use this preparation for women, recommending that the dose be a quarter of a packet applied daily to the abdominal wall. AndroGel is available in 2.5 g and 5 g sachets. This is of course an 'off-label' use, as the drug is intended for male usage.

Recent research has started to focus on loss of DHEA as a cause of decreased libido in women. DHEA levels certainly do fall, in general from the thirties onward. There has been some research showing that replacement of DHEA can increase a sense of well-being and libido. DHEA levels can be measured at most laboratories, and these levels can be followed in order to monitor replacement therapy. Again, some practitioners will start a low dose of DHEA empirically, without checking existing levels.

DHEA is available over the counter. For many years, one had to buy this substance at health-food stores. Because of its increased popularity, you can now buy it at many pharmacies as well. Because this is a non-prescription substance (and non-FDA-regulated), you need to recommend that your patient should only purchase a reputable brand. Check with your local pharmacist and a reliable health-food store so that you can recommend their reliable brands. Many practitioners feel that in general the Schiff brand is reliable. Although insurance companies will not cover DHEA therapy, it is exceptionally inexpensive, amounting to a cost of a few cents a day.

Starting doses are usually 25 to 50 mg daily. Again, as with testosterone preparations, encourage the woman to be patient, and to wait 3 months for results. If at that point she has not noted an improvement, you can measure her DHEA level and see if her dose needs to be adjusted. Of course it is possible that the DHEA may not help at all.

There is much less literature showing an improvement in libido with most other alternative treatments. Although there is some discussion of the use of the herb yohimbe for libido, there are really very few data to support its use. Another approach is the use of creams, designed for application to the vulva, containing the amino acid arginine (e.g. ArginMax®), which supposedly work by making nitric oxide more available. There are two provisos with regard to use of these topicals. First, arginine is reported to potentially exacerbate herpes, so it is not recommended for women with a history of herpes. Secondly, some of the creams also contain menthol or related substances which may irritate sensitive vulvar tissue.

As discussed above, some practitioners have tried sildenafil (Viagra) in women experimentally, and have obtained a mixed response. As most women of this age do not have significant cardiac disease which would preclude the use of the drug, it is a reasonable approach, particularly if poor orgasmic response has been an issue.

There are some non-medicinal approaches to loss of libido. The FDA has approved a device called the Eros CSD™ (clitoral stimulation device), which consists of a small manually controlled vacuum generator that is attached to tubing which ends in a cup that fits around the clitoris. The woman can use this device several times a week. The principle is that by generating a mini-vacuum at the clitoris, blood flow to the clitoris and vulva will be increased and thus enhance sexual responsiveness. The device may also be used just prior to intercourse.

This device has also been shown to be helpful in women who have undergone radical pelvic surgery (e.g. for cervical cancer), as a result of which blood flow to the pelvis in general may have been diminished.

Although the device does cost several hundred dollars, some insurance companies will cover its cost because it is used to treat female sexual dysfunction (Viagra is fairly expensive as well, and if a company covers male sexual dysfunction, many are afraid of suits for non-coverage of female sexual dysfunction). The patient will need a prescription from her healthcare provider.

To summarize, decreased sexual interest and responsiveness are among the most common issues for peri- and postmenopausal women. The evaluation is complex, but many approaches to therapy exist, and sexual counseling can always be a valuable adjunct to any medical approaches.

Vaginal dryness

Unlike hot flashes, which tend to get better over time, the progressive loss of estrogen through the peri- and postmenopause unfortunately tends to cause increasing problems with vaginal atrophy. Not all women are bothered by atrophy. Of course, overweight women will have peripheral production of estrogen, which may be sufficient to maintain vaginal lubrication. Usage of the vagina by regular sexual activity does tend to promote more pelvic blood flow, so the old adage (which your patients have heard) 'Use it or lose it' does have some truth to it.

For many women, the vaginal dryness is only an issue when they have intercourse, and they will find that a short-acting lubricant, available over the counter, is all they need. Common brands are K-Y Jelly® and Astroglide®. Discourage your patient from trying the old remedy Vaseline, because it seldom provides appropriate lubrication.

However, for many women the atrophic changes are more bothersome. They may experience recurrent vaginitis, or they may find that a simple lubricant does not help their painful intercourse. As more women are stopping their systemic HRT (or not initiating it in the first place), atrophic complaints are becoming more prevalent. And because many women are reluctant to complain of vaginal discomfort, during your annual examination of your postmenopausal patient you should specifically ask her about vaginal comfort.

Fortunately, atrophic vaginitis is fairly straightforward to treat, and multiple products are now available for therapy. The traditional standard therapies are vaginal estrogen creams. A variety of products are available, notably estradiol (Estrace) and conjugated equine estrogens (Premarin) creams. These are prescription drugs which are sold in a tube with an applicator. Woman can use 1 to 2 g of the preparation, which they place intravaginally before bedtime. Most women end up using an application two to three times per week. We encourage our patients to adjust use of the cream according to their symptomatology.

There is systemic absorption from vaginal creams, but it is relatively minor. Because endometrial hyperplasia is not seen with cream use, most gynecologists do not recommend systemic progestin withdrawal concomitant with vaginal estrogen use. Some conservative gynecologists will ask their patients to withdraw to progestins every 3 or 4 months if they are using a vaginal cream frequently. Because of the systemic absorption, some oncologists will not allow their breast cancer patients to use vaginal estrogens. This is obviously a major problem. If a young woman with breast cancer has to undergo chemotherapy, her ovaries usually cease to function, at least temporarily. These women will usually have significant atrophic symptoms, making them even more uncomfortable. The pros and cons of the therapy should therefore be considered.

More recently, a product called the Estring® has become available. This is a silicone ring which can be described to your patients as looking similar to the ring of a small contraceptive diaphragm, without the cup. It is combined with estradiol, and provides a chronic slow release of estrogen to the vaginal mucosa. The ring does elevate systemic estradiol levels for the first day that it is placed. However, shortly thereafter the blood estradiol levels fall significantly, basically back to the pre-insertion range. The ring can remain in place for 3 months, and the patient can then change it herself (or if she is unable to do so, her partner can be shown how to do this, or the occasional patient will need to have it changed by her healthcare provider). The ring is fairly unobtrusive (our patients and their partners say that they cannot feel it). Many oncologists are happier with the ring as a vaginal estrogen delivery system, because of the lower systemic levels that are reported.

Vagifem® vaginal tablets are small tablets of estradiol which can be placed vaginally to relieve atrophic symptoms. They are supplied with a vaginal applicator which is used to place the tablet high up in the vaginal vault. These tablets should be placed before bedtime, and will then dissolve. As with creams, you should explain that these products are not lubricants for intercourse, and that they should be used on a non-intercourse night. Of course, women who still require extra lubrication can use K-Y jelly or Astroglide as well.

Vagifem tablets seem to give less elevation of the serum estradiol levels, and may therefore also be preferable to creams for breast cancer patients. However, most of the time use of the various products will really depend on patient preference. For some women, the Estring is excellent, because they then only have to think about vaginal therapy once every 3 months. However, some women feel anxious about anything remaining in their body, and prefer a therapy that can be inserted on an 'as-needed' basis.

Some women prefer the feel of the vaginal creams, whereas other women find them messy and prefer the vaginal tablets, which tend to 'drip' less. Some women have atrophic symptoms of the vulva, and for these patients the cream is needed for their external anatomy. Other women will use the tablets in the vagina, and apply creams externally.

Unfortunately, these products are relatively expensive. We encourage our patients to shop around at different pharmacies and pharmacy services to find the least expensive location.

Of course, as with all estrogenic substances, some patients are unwilling even to consider any vaginal estrogens. For these women, long-acting vaginal lubricants (e.g. Replens® or Silken Glide®) are available which are placed into the vagina several times a week for relief of atrophic symptoms.

Some botanical lubricants are available. In Europe, a preparation called Phyto Soya® vaginal cream is available and is quite popular, but this particular preparation is unavailable in the USA at present. Other botanical lubricants are available and may be helpful. The vaginal mucosa is of course among the most sensitive tissues in the body, and therefore any substance can irritate it (some women are sensitive to the base in which the Estrace and Premarin products are dissolved). Therefore if your patient's vaginal complaints seem to be getting worse, not better, consider the possibility of skin irritation, and suggest an alternative product.

There is no contraindication to the concomitant use of SERMs and vaginal estrogens, so if your patient is taking raloxifene for protection against osteoporosis, there is no reason why she cannot use vaginal estrogen preparations to relieve atrophic symptoms.

Urinary symptoms

Many perimenopausal women complain for the first time in their lives of bladder problems. They may experience urinary tract infections or incontinence. Often they will end up being referred to a urologist, and they will undergo a significant work-up for a problem that could be easy to treat, as some urologists do not consider the possibility of menopausally related issues causing bladder problems.

For almost any urinary symptom, you should always start with a urinalysis and urine culture. Diabetes is now appearing in our population in epidemic proportions, and a urinalysis showing glycosuria requires further work-up. An infection in any woman requires therapy, and ideally a follow-up culture to make sure that her bacteriuria has cleared.

You should then inquire about any vaginal atrophic symptoms and perform a pelvic examination. We explain to our patients that their bladder arises embryologically from the same tissue as does their vagina, and that it possesses similar estrogen receptors. Therefore it is not surprising that women can present with symptoms related to bladder atrophic changes. In a woman with recurrent urinary tract infections, a dose of vaginal estrogens (see above) once or twice a week may be all that she requires to prevent further infections. Some women will experience urinary symptoms such as frequency, urgency and nocturia, even without infections, just related to atrophic symptoms. Vaginal estrogens, because of their absorption to the neighboring bladder, may resolve these symptoms for the patient. Of course, if she has other indications for systemic HRT, the latter should also resolve her bladder symptoms.

Incontinence is a more complicated phenomenon. Any woman who presents with leakage of urine needs to have a good history taken. Does leakage occur on coughing, sneezing or exercise? This is more commonly seen with anatomic stress incontinence. Does the woman feel that she has to get to the bathroom in a hurry? Does she leak whenever she thinks about urinating? Does she feel the need to urinate frequently? These symptoms are more common with so-called urge incontinence, or detrusor dyssynergia. Many women present with a mixed picture.

To define the patterns clearly, the patient should undergo cystometric testing in order to measure urine volumes, to ascertain at what filling point she leaks and to demonstrate whether she leaks with increased abdominal pressure. Many gynecologists can now perform these tests in their offices, as they have the appropriate equipment. Almost all urologists can perform these tests, and all urogynecologists can do so. If the patient undergoes cystometric testing, you can definitively tell her exactly which pattern she has, and manage her complaints more specifically.

However, many patients do not want to undergo these tests, and prefer to try some therapies empirically, However, if these therapies fail, testing will be helpful. The role of estrogen in the treatment of incontinence is controversial. For many years, gynecologists assumed that estrogen therapy, administered either systemically or topically, would improve both stress and urge incontinence. However, studies began to appear in the 1980s which did not show any improvement in symptoms. In the HERS trial, women on estrogen experienced more problems with incontinence, and in the Multiple Outcomes of Raloxifene Evaluation (MORE) trial of extended raloxifene use, women on raloxifene had fewer problems with stress incontinence than did the control group.

Nonetheless, many gynecologists still start a woman suffering from incontinence on either vaginal or systemic estrogens. It is certainly reasonable to try this intervention, to see whether the patient will improve.

Concomitantly, all women should be encouraged to do Kegel's exercises (squeezing of the pelvic floor muscles). Although these exercises were originally thought to help only anatomic stress incontinence, recent studies have shown that women with urge incontinence may also benefit from them. You can check your patient during her pelvic examination to see whether she is doing her exercises correctly (simply ask the patient to contract her vaginal muscles around your fingers during a digital examination).

Encourage your patient to do as many Kegel's exercises as she can during the day. We encourage our patients to put a sign on the dashboard of their car, to remind them to do Kegel's while they are stopped at stoplights, or in traffic. Another time they could do them is while pumping gas.

Many physical therapists are now trained in pelvic floor exercises. You can refer your patient to such a therapist, who may be able to improve your patient's techniques and her pelvic floor strength. Most physical therapists will incorporate biofeedback techniques as well.

Weight is also a major factor here. Weight loss will almost always improve incontinence. Of course, if a patient is contemplating any surgical procedure for incontinence, one of the major causes of surgical failure is obesity. Therefore weight loss will either remove the patient's need for surgical intervention or, if she still requires surgery, it will significantly improve the chances of success.

For the patient for whom weight loss, Kegel's exercises and estrogen therapy have failed, other pharmacological interventions for incontinence are available. For the patient with urge incontinence, the old standard therapy was oxybutinin (Ditropan®). The actions of oxybutinin are anticholinergic, and although it often worked well for urge incontinence, the side-effects of dry mouth and constipation were often more unpleasant for the patient than the incontinence. However, a newer extended-release product is available, and with this XL product, the side-effects have been reduced.

Tolterodine (Detrol®) was developed more recently. Its activity is also anticholinergic, but it has less of a dry-mouth effect. It is also available in a long-acting form. The major contraindication of Ditropan and Detrol is uncontrolled narrow-angle glaucoma. These drugs will act fairly quickly, so that in a matter of a few days to weeks your patients' responses can be clearly seen.

Although the approach to urge incontinence is primarily pharmacological, the approach to stress incontinence has traditionally been surgical or mechanical (in the form of pessaries). However, a product for stress incontinence will shortly be available in the USA. Duloxetine®, a relative of venlafaxine, an SSRI and SNRI antidepressant, has been shown to be effective in contracting pelvic floor muscles, thereby producing a decrease in stress incontinence in many women. It also has antidepressant effects and therefore, particularly if the patient has problems with depression and stress incontinence, it may be an ideal drug. It should be available shortly.

Pessaries have been available for many years. Many younger practitioners have never seen a pessary. This is a rubber or plastic gadget which is available in many shapes, from rings to cubes to dishes, which are designed to fit in the vagina and support the pelvic floor, and by exerting pressure on the urethra to stop leakage of urine. Many women are quite comfortable using them and become adept at inserting and removing them themselves. For the woman who does not wish to undergo surgery, pessaries may be an ideal solution. For women who develop mild incontinence, particularly with exercise, insertion of a vaginal tampon prior to exercise may relieve their symptoms.

For women who are extremely poor surgical candidates, pessaries can also be very useful. These women, who are often elderly and have significant prolapse as well as incontinence, will usually be unable to remove these pessaries on their own, and will require a check-up by the practitioner every 3 or 4 months to remove the pessary and cleanse the vagina.

For younger women with true stress incontinence for whom more conservative therapy has failed, surgical intervention can be quite helpful. Traditional bladder suspension procedures have been performed for many years. Many urogynecologists are now using the tension-free vaginal tapes to suspend the bladder and urethra. The advantages of this procedure are that it is performed on an outpatient basis, with relatively quick recuperation. The initial success data are good, but obviously long-term data are not yet available.

Again, as many women are embarrassed about discussing incontinence, if you feel that this is an issue for your patient, raise it with her, and reassure her that this is an extremely common problem. Encourage her to think about interventions.

Weight gain

Weight gain is another controversial issue in menopause management. Many experts believe that women gain weight as they age, and that the gain which women experience at menopause is just an aging phenomenon and is not related to a lack of hormones. Other studies have suggested a modest weight gain, of 5 to 8 pounds, related to menopause itself. Certainly if your patient reports that she has gained 30 pounds over the last year, and she attributes it all to the menopause, you can assure her that such an explanation is extremely unlikely.

Indeed, many women who might otherwise want to take HRT for relief of menopausal symptoms have been reluctant to start therapy because they are anxious that it will lead to weight gain. You can reassure them that estrogen can cause a modest amount of fluid retention, which will cease with estrogen administration, but that this should amount to a weight gain of 2 to 3 pounds at most. Long-term trials such as the Postmenopausal Estrogen/Progestin Interventions (PEPI) trial showed that long-term HRT users actually lost a very small amount of weight, so long-term therapy does not appear to add pounds.

Given that estrogen therapy does not seem to alter the weight gain at menopause substantially, theories have arisen as to the actual cause of the weight gain. Some have hypothesized that growth hormone levels decrease, leading to a slowing of the basal metabolic rate. Others suggest that post-menopausal women are less active and maintain less muscle mass because of this decreased activity. This decrease in lean body mass also leads to a lower caloric requirement, so if one maintains the same caloric intake as before, one will gain weight.

As thyroid disease becomes more prevalent with increasing age, it is quite appropriate to test for hypothyroidism at this point (it is currently recommended as a screening test for all 50-year-olds, in any case). If you see an elevated TSH level, institution of thyroid replacement therapy is indicated and very straightforward.

Unfortunately, most of the time the TSH level is normal, and your patient is just unhappy that she is gaining weight for whatever reason, menopause or not. As we explain to our patients, there is no simple pill to swallow to make them stay slim. The standard therapy is still the best – a low-calorie diet and plenty of exercise.

Many patients will do better with an organized diet. Seeing a registered dietitian may be the answer for your patient. Programs such as Weight Watchers or TOPS (Take Off Pounds Sensibly) may be helpful for patients who do better with a group program. They must view this as a lifelong project, not a short-term answer. Become acquainted with the resources available in your area, to whom you can refer your patients.

With a sensible diet, perimenopausal and postmenopausal women all need an exercise regime. This may just be walking regularly. Two miles a day is an excellent goal, and will help your patient not only to maintain her weight, but also to decrease her risks of osteoporosis, cardiac disease and probably even breast cancer. If she is a gym person, encourage her to go regularly, at least three or four times a week, and encourage her to work out for at least 30 to 45 min at a time. A national chain of gyms, called Curves for Women, is very popular in our area, and has a relatively efficient prescribed workout.

We also encourage all healthcare providers to be visible leaders in physical fitness in their towns. All providers should be physically fit, because otherwise we lack credibility recommending things to our patients that we are unwilling to do ourselves. Go to the gyms that your patients go to, and become a role model. If your town has road races, help to sponsor them, and then participate in them. Even the last person to cross the finishing line has done great exercise, and if you participate, you show that you mean what you recommend.

As we discuss the different medical problems that our patients face during the menopause in subsequent chapters, remember that exercise helps to prevent almost all of these problems.

CONTRACEPTION AND SEXUALLY TRANSMITTED DISEASES

Contraception

Although it is a well-known fact that fertility declines with age, we need to remind all of our patients that until they go for a full year without a menstrual period, they need to practice contraception. One of the authors has personally assisted two 47-year-olds in giving birth, both of whom were convinced that their skipped menses were secondary to menopause, not to pregnancy (and one of whom did not present until 20 weeks' gestation, when her abdomen became somewhat more protuberant; the author also had to personally arrange for her amniocentesis that day, as the Down's risk at these older ages is astronomical).

Some experts will recommend determining the patient's FSH level. As we have previously discussed, FSH levels can be very deceptive. Someone may have a significantly elevated FSH level, and then 2 months later have a completely normal one. Therefore if you are going to rely on an FSH level to tell a patient that she does not require contraception, you should repeat the test after another 2 or 3 months, to make sure that the level is consistently elevated.

The contraceptive benefit of birth control pills is obvious, in that they provide both hormonal control of symptoms and contraception. Such a dual-purpose intervention can be particularly helpful for your patient who may have been relying on the rhythm method, but who can no longer do so given her likely menstrual irregularity.

If a women needs contraception and is not an oral contraceptive candidate, she may be permitted to rely on less effective methods. Although you would not encourage a teenager to rely on contraceptive foams or the sponge alone, a perimenopausal woman's fertility is sufficiently reduced that the 90% reliability of such a method should be adequate.

Another promising new option would be a progestin-containing intrauterine device (IUD), such as Mirena®. Active for 5 years, the progestin released by the IUD is sufficient to protect the endometrium, if the patient wanted to take estrogen replacement therapy. Thus she would be obtaining contraception and hormonal benefit concurrently.

Sexually transmitted diseases

Although the risk of conception disappears at menopause, the risk of sexually transmitted diseases (STDs) does not. We have seen patients plagued by herpes that was acquired postmenopausally. Sometimes such symptoms can be exacerbated by the atrophic changes that the woman may be experiencing, making therapy quite challenging.

Postmenopausal women often acquire new partners, either after their partner dies or after they divorce. These women need to be reminded that they are at risk of all STDs, and that although they do not need to worry about a pregnancy, they need to worry about infectious agents. Encourage all of your patients to use a condom when becoming involved in any new relationship, and to continue condom use until their partner has been tested for HIV at the very minimum, and they are certain that this relationship is mutually monogamous.

SPECIAL NEEDS PATIENTS: WOMEN AFTER HYSTERECTOMY

The patient with a bilateral salpingoophorectomy

We need to consider women who have had a hysterectomy as a separate group. Gynecologists are certainly removing ovaries less frequently now than they did many years ago. However, there are still certain patients who will need oophorectomies, including women with severe endometriosis or pelvic inflammatory disease, women who have a history of familial ovarian cancer or are BRCA-positive, and women who request prophylactic oophorectomy at the time of their hysterectomy.

Assuming that they are premenopausal, these patients will need hormonal intervention shortly after surgery in order to avoid severe symptomatology. Many physicians will place an estrogen patch on these women either at the time of surgery or the next day. Most of these women will acutely need higher doses of estrogen than a typical non-surgical patient, as they have an acute loss of ovarian function. We tell our patients that we will start at a moderate dose rather than a low dose, and taper down slowly. However, we always caution them to call us if they start to develop severe flashing, night sweats or insomnia, as they may need more estrogen than we anticipated. If we are using a patch, we will usually start with a 0.1 mg/day patch. If we are starting with oral estrogens (and again discuss the woman's preference pre-operatively), we will start with 2 mg of estradiol or 1.25 mg of conjugated estrogens.

On the longer-term basis, you need to discuss with these patients the possibility of testosterone replacement. Remind the woman that her ovaries were making testosterone as well as estrogen, and that testosterone is also a female hormone. Many practitioners do not routinely start their post-oophorectomy patients on testosterone as well as estrogen, but you need to have a low threshold for adding testosterone if the patient complains of low libido or loss of energy.

Indeed, because of testosterone issues some reproductive endocrinologists do not recommend routine bilateral salpingoophorectomy at the time of a postmenopausal hysterectomy. They state that although the ovaries are not making estrogen, they are still (if the operation is performed reasonably soon after the menopause) making substantial amounts of androgens, and that oophorectomy is undesirable because it will remove valuable hormones. Most gynecologic oncologists would disagree, and advocate oophorectomy and testosterone replacement as needed.

There is also currently considerable controversy over the health value of replacing estrogens in younger women after oophorectomy. There is a considerable body of literature from many years ago demonstrating that if young women who are deprived of ovarian function are not given estrogen, their rates of atherosclerotic heart disease and osteoporosis skyrocket, with a seven-fold increase in coronary heart disease in women who have their ovaries removed before the age of 35 years. Given the current anti-estrogen climate, these women need considerable counseling. We think it is helpful to point out to them that had they not had their ovaries removed, their own levels of estrogen production would be substantially higher than the amount of estrogen we are giving them, and that they therefore need not be anxious about taking HRT.

The patient who has a hysterectomy without an oophorectomy

Even if you leave the ovaries in place, many women will acutely complain of hot flashes for several weeks after a hysterectomy. Many practitioners assume that this is due to blood flow changes within the pelvis. Estrogen replacement therapy usually works in this situation, and we titrate the dose to the patient's needs. We offer them the choice of pill or patch, and usually start with a relatively low dose (1 mg of estradiol or a 0.05 mg/day patch) and increase the doses until the symptoms subside. We explain to the patient that we will usually be able to withdraw the estrogen within a month or two, and she will be fine.

There is some literature to suggest that women who have had hysterectomies do undergo an earlier menopause. Again this is presumed to be due to alterations in pelvic blood flow, with decreasing ovarian blood supply. This literature suggests as much as a 2-year acceleration in loss of ovarian function.

Given that these women are not having periods, it is often difficult to assess when they are menopausal. One must listen to their accounts of their symptoms, and assess their estrogen levels by looking at the vaginal tissue at their examination. This scenario is one of the few in which determining FSH and estradiol levels will help you considerably.

In post-hysterectomy patients it is of course easier to use hormonal therapy for replacement. As you do not have to consider progestins and their side-effects, it is straightforward to balance the doses of estrogen. At the time of publication of this book, the post-hysterectomy arm of the WHI is still ongoing. Given the current climate, it makes sense to keep these women on the lowest dose that will alleviate their symptoms.

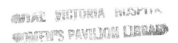

3

Menopause: disease states

OSTEOPOROSIS

When educated women think of the menopause, they think of osteoporosis. Any knowledgeable woman will worry about her likelihood of losing bone, fracturing her hip and ending up immobile in a nursing home. It is our job to help to prevent exactly this scenario. Remember that 20% of women who sustain a hip fracture die within the next year.

Defined as bone loss and loss of bone architecture (the latter cannot be clinically measured) which increases fracture risk, osteoporosis can be quantified by measuring bone mineral density with a dual-energy X-ray absorptiometry (DEXA) scan. The more energy a tissue absorbs, the denser it is, and this principle has been put to good use in this test. One of the major controversies in menopause management concerns who should be tested for bone density using this rather expensive test. You can assure your patient that this test is very easy – it is performed just like a standard X-ray, taking a picture of the hip and the spine, and in some instances the forearm. It is significantly less uncomfortable than a mammogram, so you can assure your patient that it will not hurt.

Your patient may ask about the less expensive ultrasound tests of the heel, which are often used as screening tests. These ultrasound examinations are quite reasonable, but are not as definitive as the DEXA scan. If a patient has a heel test which shows osteoporosis, she should go on to have a DEXA scan so that her bone loss can be accurately quantified and monitored. However, if her ultrasound test is normal, this is not a guarantee that she does not have osteoporosis. Many women will have a normal ultrasound test but have significant bone loss on the more definitive DEXA scan. Therefore if she is a high-risk patient, do encourage her to obtain a DEXA scan.

Some women may have heard about measurement of serum or urinary biochemical markers for bone turnover. Bone experts will use these clinically

Table 2 Risk factors for osteoporosis

Familial history of osteoporosis and fractures
Personal history of non-traumatic fractures
Advancing age
Caucasian or Asian descent
Being fair skinned
A small frame or thinness
Late puberty, early menopause (natural or medically/surgically induced)
Removal of ovaries before the age of 45 years
Significant episodes of exercise- or weight-loss-induced amenorrhea
Smoking
Sedentary lifestyle
No children
Excessive alcohol consumption
Inadequate dairy/calcium intake
Disease medications (i.e., steroids, anticonvulsants, thyroid hormone)
Diabetes
Hypoglycemia
Kidney or liver disease
Thyroid disease
Anorexia or excessive dieting

to measure a response to therapy, or occasionally to ascertain why a woman might have excessive bone loss. However, they are rarely used as a screening test, although they are widely used in research protocols.

Of course, the least expensive test is an annual height measurement. Your medical assistant can easily obtain a height measurement together with the annual weight and blood pressure test (also a height measurement counts as a vital sign, when HMOs review your charts to make sure that you are monitoring your patients closely enough). Many adults will lose an inch or one and a half inches from peak height. However, a loss of more than 4 cm or so requires evaluation.

One of the few areas of agreement in the business is that all women should have a test by the time they reach the age of 65 years. However, there is little agreement as to who should have one, and exactly when, before that time.

Many women like to have a test done as they reach menopause. This is certainly reasonable, as they will then know whether they are entering a high-risk time with good bones. There are multiple risk factors for bone loss, the most common of which are listed in Table 2. If your patient has several of these risk factors, a bone density test is warranted. Even if she only has some degree of bone loss, but not severe bone loss (usually defined as osteopenia), we find that a bone density test makes the patient much more

50

aware of bone health. Many women are then much more likely to follow guidelines for better bone health, even if they do not need pharmacological intervention.

Of course, women should always do everything they can to promote healthier bones. However, sometimes just knowing that a DEXA scan has shown that her bone structure is not spectacular will make a woman much more willing to do the right things for her bones. One of the ways in which we try to enhance compliance with a healthy regime is by playing on the patient's fears. This may sound like an 'evil' thing to do, but if you significantly improve her health as a result, you are doing the right thing. For example, if the patient's mother has just been placed in a nursing home because of a hip fracture, you can remind her that she does not want to end up like her mother. And every time you see that patient for her annual examination, you should ask how her mother is doing after her hip fracture.

What are the right things for such a woman's bones? One of the first things you can encourage her to do is to stop smoking. Smoking does lead to premature ovarian failure (by about 2 years), so in general a smoker will enter a low-estrogen state 2 years earlier than a non-smoker, which increases bone loss. Persistent smoking promotes osteroporosis.

Encourage adequate calcium intake, as almost all women need calcium. One of the traditional concerns is that if a woman has a history of calcium kidney stones, she will increase her likelihood of developing more stones if she increases her calcium intake. This is not so. Studies have shown that an intake of up to 1500 mg of calcium per day does not increase renal stone formation.

How much calcium should your patient be taking in daily? An easy guideline is that if she is premenopausal or taking HRT, 1000 mg a day is good. If she is postmenopausal and not on HRT, she should be taking in 1500 mg a day. The other important point is to encourage her not to take all her calcium at once. Recent studies have shown that a woman can only absorb about 500 mg of calcium at any one meal, so that any amount she ingests above this level is not being absorbed. For example, any cereal advertisement she sees that says she will obtain 100% of her daily calcium requirement by eating brand X cereal at breakfast is false advertising – it may contain 100% of her daily requirement, but she will be unlikely to absorb it.

You should first assess the woman's calcium intake from food. The mainstay of calcium intake consists of dairy products. An 8-ounce glass of milk (whole or skimmed), an 8-ounce cup of yogurt and a 1-ounce slice of hard cheese each contain approximately 300 mg of calcium. The only dairy product which is actually not calcium rich is cottage cheese. Many women consume considerable amounts of cottage cheese because it is relatively low in calories, so encourage them to eat low-fat hard cheese instead.

The only other major calcium source in foods is broccoli. A cup of broccoli will also provide about 300 mg of calcium (an easy number to remember). Kale is the second-best vegetable, and most others lag fairly far behind. You have to eat four bags of spinach in order to ingest 300 mg of calcium – that is a lot of spinach. Certain other foods (such as sardines that still contain the bones) are fine, but very few women eat enough of these to benefit their daily intake.

This leads on to the issue of augmenting dietary intake with calcium supplements, which is an area fraught with controversy. Some experts say that you need calcium with magnesium, or that you need calcium citrate, or they discourage you from taking Tums® products. We think the most important thing is to achieve compliance with whatever regime is acceptable to your patient. The only people who really have to take calcium citrate preparations are those with decreased gastric acid production, such as individuals with true pernicious anemia.

In general, our advice to our patients to enhance compliance is to buy whatever brand of calcium agrees best with their gastrointestinal tracts and is cheapest. Many women find calcium constipating, and they may need to try several types in order to find the least constipating one. Furthermore, some brands are significantly more expensive than others. Tums in general are fairly cheap, and are well tolerated. One famous osteoporosis physician ends his talks by saying 'I tell all my patients to chew one extra-strength Tums for dessert at every meal'.

One recently marketed form of calcium consists of the chewable preparations. The first on the market was a 'candy' called Viactiv®, which is marketed as an individually wrapped piece. These candies come in multiple flavors, including chocolate, and most people find them fairly pleasant to ingest. They only contain 20 calories, and each piece contains 500 mg of calcium and 100 units of vitamin D. Therefore for women who complain that they cannot take calcium because they call the traditional pills 'horse pills' which they cannot swallow, this is a good way to supplement their calcium intake.

Some of the preparations also contain vitamin D, while others do not. If your patient is obtaining her calcium from non-dairy sources, she will need vitamin D supplementation. Current daily recommendations are 400 units of vitamin D for women under the age of 65 years, and 600 units for those over 65 years. Almost all multivitamin preparations that are sold in the USA contain 400 units of vitamin D, so if your patient is concerned about whether she is getting enough vitamin D, ask her if she takes a multivitamin, and to check the side of the bottle to make sure that it contains vitamin D.

All women who are capable of doing weight-bearing exercise should be encouraged to do so. The way we describe it to patients is 'driving the calcium into the bone'. Basically almost all exercise is good, except for swimming and aquatic-based programs, which are excellent for cardiovascular fitness and joint mobility but do not have an effect on bone, so just encourage those women to add some weight-bearing exercise. Of course you will want to encourage good exercise regimes for cardiovascular fitness as well. Moreover, being fit will decrease the likelihood of falls later on, and by preventing falls you will have a profound impact on fracture rates as well.

When is pharmacological intervention appropriate?

Again this is a controversial topic. If a woman has established osteoporosis, all practitioners would agree that drug therapy is needed. If she has experienced an osteoporotic fracture, she requires intervention, because the greatest risk factor for developing a new fracture is a previous fracture. If a woman has significant osteopenia and also has other significant risk factors, most experts would agree that she should receive medication. If for some reason you have measured her estradiol level and found it to be extremely low (< 5 pg/ml), this patient will be at increased risk of fracture and will require more aggressive therapy.

However, there is less consensus of opinion on women without these precise conditions, primarily the patient with moderate osteopenia. Some authors argue that some women have less bone mass than others, and just because a patient has a somewhat lower bone mass than others does not mandate medical intervention beyond optimizing lifestyle issues. Others are concerned that these women are at higher risk, and that it is better to prevent further bone loss before it occurs. Similarly, there is no consensus on how often to repeat a study, with or without pharmacological intervention. Most menopause physicians would tend to repeat a bone density scan on these women every 2 to 3 years.

Some patients will obsess about their bone density testing, and particularly if they have osteoporosis or significant osteopenia they may want to have a test repeated in 6 months. Such a test would seldom be worthwhile, as the standard error of interpretation of the test would be greater than any significant change that one would see. Try to encourage such patients to wait at

Table 3 Medications for osteoporosis therapy

Medication	Therapeutic dose	Prophylactic dose
Raloxifene (Evista®)	60 mg daily	60 mg daily
Alendronate (Fosamax®)	10 mg daily	5 mg daily
	70 mg weekly	35 mg weekly
Risedronate (Actonel®)	5 mg daily	5 mg daily
	35 mg weekly	35 mg weekly
Calcitonin nasal spray (Miacalcin®)	200 IU daily (one spray intranasally)	not indicated

least a year before repeating the test (also very few insurers would reimburse them for a test performed after less than a 1-year interval).

What medications should be used for osteoporosis therapy?

Fortunately we live in an era of multiple options for interventions. Of course one should always take the whole patient into account when prescribing any medication, and bone therapy really should be individualized, taking into account the side-benefits (or lack of them) of the intervention, and the side-effects of the drug. And no matter what drug intervention you prescribe, you need to emphasize that the patient must concomitantly make the appropriate lifestyle modifications described above.

For the patient who is menopausal and experiencing significant problems with hot flashes, insomnia and other symptoms due to her lack of estrogen, HRT would be the first choice, assuming that she wanted hormonal intervention. You would repeat the bone density test in a year or two, and reassess her situation with the bone response. At that point you might try to taper the patient off HRT and see how she felt. If she felt well off therapy, you might then choose an alternative bone preservation option.

For the patient with minimal or no menopausal symptomatology, there are several options (see Table 3). Raloxifene (Evista®) is a selective estrogen receptor modulator that is indicated for both osteoporosis prevention and therapy. It acts like estrogen to prevent resorption of bone. At the level of the breast it acts as an estrogen blocker, and in several trials of raloxifene use, breast cancer occurrence rates were substantially reduced in women who were taking the drug. These reduction rates were comparable to those seen with the use of tamoxifen in breast cancer prevention models, leading to the initiation of the STAR (Study of Tamoxifen and Raloxifene) trial to see a head-to-head comparison of the breast cancer protection offered by the two drugs. The results of this study will not be available for several years. However, if your patient is also at significant risk for development of breast cancer (e.g. due to a strong family history and low parity), raloxifene offers the side-benefit of a possible reduction in breast cancer risk.

Tamoxifen does act as a bone-protective agent. As we explain to patients, tamoxifen is a breast-protective drug that helps to protect the bone, whereas raloxifene is a bone-protective drug that may help to protect the breast. However, we must remember that many breast cancer patients are currently being treated with aromatase inhibitors, which may actually increase the fracture risk, so these women must be evaluated for bone loss and treated appropriately with additional therapy as necessary.

Raloxifene does not stimulate the endometrium, which gives it an advantage over tamoxifen, which does. If the STAR trial shows that raloxifene is as effective as tamoxifen for breast cancer protection, then for the woman who is at risk for endometrial carcinoma, raloxifene would have an advantage.

Raloxifene also induces a favorable lipid profile. In several studies, total cholesterol and low-density lipoprotein (LDL) levels have been lowered in users, as have homocysteine levels. There is currently an ongoing study called the RUTH (Raloxifene Use in the Heart) study which is looking at the incidence of cardiovascular disease in high-risk patients who are using raloxifene. It is a prospective double-blind randomized control trial, and its results will not be available for several years.

Raloxifene can be taken at any time of the day, with or without meals, and it is taken on a daily basis. The major health drawback of this drug is that, like estrogen, it increases the risk of thrombophlebitis. As with estrogen, the highest incidence of clotting disorders is seen during the first 6 months of therapy. If a woman has been on estrogen previously and has not had phlebitis, she is unlikely to develop it *de novo* from raloxifene.

Raloxifene use can precipitate hot flashes. Some authors feel that introducing the drug on an every-other-day basis can minimize these symptoms. We also always recommend to our patients who are stopping estrogen and switching to raloxifene for osteoporosis therapy that they stay off everything for a month, so that we can see whether they develop hot flashes from merely being off the estrogen, rather than secondary to raloxifene use. A recent study has actually shown that the majority of women who develop hot flashes with estrogen withdrawal will develop them within 2 months, but a few will develop some hot flashes over a 3-month period. Therefore some women who think that their flashes are due to raloxifene are still developing flashes as a result of estrogen withdrawal. A few patients may also complain of leg cramps (unrelated to any phlebitis).

The other major category of drugs for osteoporosis prevention and therapy consists of the bisphosphonates alendronate (Fosamax®) and risedronate (Actonel®). They also prevent bone resorption and are non-hormonal. One of the major advantages of both medications is that they can be taken once a week. We encourage our patients to link the use of this medication to a weekly morning activity, such as going to church on Sunday.

The major point to consider with bisphosphonate use is exactly how to take the medication. Your patient should be advised to take the medication first thing in the morning with a glass of water. She should then stay upright and not lie down, and eat her breakfast half an hour later. This regime was occasionally a nuisance for women when they had to take the medication daily. However, with a once-a-week dosing schedule, it is not a problem for most women. Nevertheless, even with this regime a few women will experience esophageal irritation, which for a few may preclude the use of the drug.

Therefore if a patient has chronic gastroesophageal reflux disease, bisphosphonates may not be the best choice. However, if your patient has a history of phlebitis, she will not be taking estrogen or raloxifene, and a bisphosphonate will be a better choice. Clearly these choices really depend significantly on other patient health issues.

Alendronate and risedronate both have significant beneficial effects on bone, and increases in bone mineral density (BMD) are seen within the first year of use. One question regularly arises with regard to interpretation of the effects of all antiresorptive therapy. Many people merely look at the BMD response of any of these agents. However, the BMD is really just a surrogate marker, just as a lipid profile is used to evaluate the risk of a myocardial infarction. What you really need to assess with any antiresorptive therapy is the following: 'Does this medication reduce the risk of fracture?'. Although all of the different therapies may show slight differences in BMD responses, all of the therapies discussed are quite effective in reducing fractures.

Another question that is often raised by compulsive patients is 'Can I take two different therapies together to get a better bone mineral density response?' (e.g. alendronate and raloxifene). We do know that the combination will increase the BMD further. However, there are no data to demonstrate that the risk of fracture is further reduced.

Calcitonin nasal spray (Miacalcin®) has been approved by the FDA for osteoporosis therapy but not prevention. It may have some effects on bone pain associated with significant osteoporosis with fractures, and some practitioners will use it with another agent for that reason. It has a small effect on BMD, and is not widely used.

Tibolone® is available in Europe but not in the USA at the time of writing. It does have significant effects on bone improvement, and as its metabolites have estrogenic, progestogenic and androgenic effects, it has been shown in some European studies to help to relieve some menopausal symptoms.

For women with advanced osteoporosis, parathyroid hormone therapy (Forteo®) has been approved by the FDA. This is not a prevention drug, nor should it be used for women with mild osteoporosis. However, for women with profound bone loss and fractures, this drug is extremely powerful. It is given as a daily injection for 18 months, and its use would then be followed by an antiresorptive agent. This medication is also very expensive, but when think- ing about the cost of an agent such as this, one must balance it against the high cost (both personal and financial) of treating a fracture. By the time a woman is using this drug, it is unlikely that her gynecologist would be in charge of monitoring her bone loss. Most of these women are under the care of an internist, with back-up from either an endocrinologist or a rheumatologist.

However, you should never assume that your menopausal patient is automatically receiving proper follow-up of her osteoporosis. Many orthopedic surgeons will treat your patient for her hip fracture, and not perform a bone density test on her, nor will they prescribe the appropriate medication. If during her annual visit your patient lets you know that she has sustained a fracture during the previous year, specifically ask her if she has had a DEXA scan since then, and if not, you should arrange it, and then follow it up with appropriate medication recommendations.

CARDIOVASCULAR DISEASES

Cardiovascular diseases are the number-one killer of women in the USA, and their incidence increases dramatically at the menopause. However, we dis- cuss them here second, as most women with significant CAD will be moni- tored by their internist or cardiologist, who will be managing their various lipid-lowering, blood-pressure-lowering and hypoglycemic agents. Women with bone loss may have fewer other complicating medical illnesses, and may be managed primarily by the caregiver who is managing their menopause.

However, the caregivers who provide primary care for women as they enter menopause have a very significant role in diagnosing those women who require cardiovascular interventions. Furthermore, many women regard the menopause as a significant life landmark, and may view this transition

Table 4   Risk factors for coronary artery disease

Advanced age
Postmenopause status (notably if menopause reached before the age of 40 years)
Oophorectomy
Family history of first heart attack in a male relative before the age of 50 years or in a female relative before the age of 60 years
African-American descent
High blood pressure
Elevated cholesterol levels
Elevated triglyceride levels
Obesity
Diabetes
Physical inactivity
Cigarette smoking
Stress
Consumption of more than three alcoholic beverages daily

time as an opportunity to make significant lifestyle changes, which can have huge cardiovascular ramifications. Although you will of course have counseled your patient to stop smoking at every visit for many years, by raising this issue at the time of the menopause, which is also a time of increased cardiovascular risk, you may reach her at a more receptive moment. You need to emphasize to the woman that smoking is itself a major risk factor for CAD (see Table 4), and that the menopause will compound that risk for her.

If your patient has not had a lipid profile done within a year after her last menstrual period, you should order one. Without estrogen, the LDL may rise and high-density lipoprotein (HDL) may fall, and you need to know by how much.

Even if the patient's lipid profile is perfect, you should encourage her to do regular aerobic exercise. Walking for 10 min, three times a day for 5 days a week will provide her with aerobic benefits (and the more the better). However, if her lipid profile is not perfect, it is particularly important to encourage her to become aerobically fit. You would like her to have a total cholesterol concentration under 200 mg/dl, with an HDL level above 55 mg/dl and triglycerides less than 150 mg/dl. If she has a significant family history of early CAD, or is diabetic, you would want those figures to be even better.

Another side-benefit of exercise would be stress reduction. Although the exact increase in risk is debated, most experts agree that stress compounds cardiovascular risk, and a regular aerobic program will help your patient to reduce her stress levels.

Again, even if she is at her ideal body weight, you still want to encourage her to eat a healthy diet. You should encourage her to eat a diet that is rich in fruit, vegetables and fish but low in animal fats. If she is overweight, you should encourage her to cut down on calories in order to try to achieve an ideal body weight. However, even if she cannot reach her ideal body weight, you can tell her that if she can manage to reduce her body weight by 10% over the next 6 months (or as soon as she can manage), she will substantially reduce her risk of atherosclerotic heart disease. Again, putting her in touch with a nutritionist or a weight reduction support group may help her significantly. Hypertensive patients need to be reminded to maintain a low-salt diet.

There is considerable controversy about the use of complementary nd alternative medicines for the prevention of heart disease. There are advocates of vitamin B, C and E supplementation, with very little proven data to endorse the use of such supplements. However, they are relatively safe if used in reasonable rather than excessive doses. If a patient will be more compliant about eating a proper diet and taking regular exercise if she is also taking reasonable doses of vitamins, we will certainly encourage her to continue her regime. Some cardiologists believe that homocysteine levels provide another marker for CAD risk. If these levels are elevated, most of these practitioners would recommend vitamin B_6 (50 mg) and folic acid (1 mg) therapeutically.

There have been some recent studies of the use of soy to prevent heart disease. NAMS has also encouraged the use of soy (this is whole soy, not isolated isoflavones in supplement form). Again, the use of soy, can be incorporated with the recommendations for a high intake of vegetables and fruits in the diet.

Many cardiologists do recommend the addition of fish-oil capsules or ground-up flaxseed oil to achieve the same levels of omega 3 fatty acids that produce the effects of the Mediterranean diet. The latter diet, as confirmed by the Lyon Heart Study, has been shown to reduce the incidence of CAD.

The use of aspirin therapy for the prevention of CAD in women is still somewhat controversial. Most cardiologists would recommend aspirin therapy as prophylaxis for women with existing disease, to prevent recurrence. However, the data on primary prevention for women are more limited, and thus controversial. Again, given that the woman with already diagnosed CAD should be followed by her cardiologist or internist, we usually recommend that our patients follow their cardiologists' recommendations with regard to medication.

For many years, healthcare providers have encouraged women to initiate HRT at menopause for the prevention of heart disease. The HERS study basically stopped the use of HRT for secondary prevention, and the American Heart Association very quickly endorsed the findings of the HERS study. The WHI has now called into question the use of HRT for primary prevention, and based on the findings of the WHI, we are not supposed to recommend hormonal therapy to prevent CAD. However, if a woman is suffering from significant menopausal symptoms, the WHI does not preclude the use of estrogen for these women. If a woman is asymptomatic, but has a worrying lipid profile, the first choice of therapy is now statin therapy.

Women with coronary risk factors have always presented a challenge for HRT. The lipid-related effects of hormones have been known for many years. Oral estrogens will lower LDL and increase HDL, but also increase triglycerides, potentially substantially. Transdermal estrogen patches do not have quite so profound an effect on lowering LDL or increasing HDL, but they do not elevate triglyceride levels. Therefore if your patient has a problem with triglycerides, or is diabetic (a group for which you want to be especially wary about triglycerides), transdermal patches are probably a better way to institute therapy than are tablets. Both oral and transdermal estrogens produce vasodilatation.

As transdermal estrogens are absorbed directly into the bloodstream, and avoid the first-pass effect on the liver, there is less stimulation of substances produced by the liver. Thus from a theoretical basis, as clotting factors are produced in the liver, the transdermal patches should have less of an effect on thrombogenesis. Although the theory is quite reasonable, there are no clinical data that confirm this theoretical principle. Again, though, if estrogen is not contraindicated, but there is some concern about thrombosis, many would recommend the patch.

Again, in line with the recommendations of the WHI, most experts would suggest the lowest dose of estrogen that would relieve the woman's symptoms. One can always titrate upward in order to achieve symptom relief.

Of course, if the patient still has a uterus, you need to add progesterone to protect against endometrial hyperplasia. And although most authors have always felt that estrogens are 'heart-friendly', most have also believed that progestins can undo a significant amount of the good done by estrogens. Estrogen raises HDL, whereas progestins will lower it, and estrogen decreases

LDL, whereas progestins will raise it. Medroxyprogesterone acetate (Provera®) has been shown to produce vascular spasm.

Thus from a cardiovascular viewpoint, you want to use the lowest possible amount of progestin for the least amount of time. For this reason, many cardiovascularly oriented gynecologists advocate using progestin therapy for 12 days every other month, on a cyclic basis, rather than daily therapy (this is one of the reasons why some gynecologists believe that the WHI failed in using continuous combined therapy).

The other major question apart from timing and duration of progestin therapy is choice of progestin. The PEPI trial used natural progesterone in one of its arms, and showed no adverse effects on lipids. Natural progesterone does not raise LDL levels in contrast to medroxyprogesterone. This is another reason why some authors believe that the WHI failed, in that they used the wrong progesterone.

For many years, natural progesterone (in a micronized form which was necessary for absorption) was only available from compounding pharmacies. However, oral micronized progesterone is now available from your local drugstore. Manufactured as Prometrium, natural micronized oral progesterone, dissolved in a peanut oil base, is available in 100 mg and 200 mg capsules. Standard dosages for cyclical withdrawal therapy would be 200 mg orally for 12 days every other month. This regime should prevent endometrial hyperplasia.

One word of advice when using natural progesterone – it can be sedating, so it is best taken before bedtime and away from food intake. However, if it does not sedate your patient, she can take it at any time of day.

Therefore if you have a patient who is significantly symptomatic, but you are concerned about her lipid profile, the combination of transdermal estrogens and natural progesterone would be the best of the currently available options.

Some new compounds are being tested. The new progestin drospirenone has some very interesting properties. Derived from the antimineralocorticoid spironolactone, it has progestational activities but also spironolactone-type activities, including lowering of blood pressure. It has been used in oral contraceptive therapy (Yasmin), and trials are ongoing for its use as a component of HRT. Some researchers have been looking specifically at its role in women with metabolic syndrome.

There is also no contraindication to the simultaneous use of HRT and statin therapy, so if your patient on statins for her lipid profile becomes menopausal and significantly symptomatic, she can be started on HRT.

COLON CANCER

The risks of colorectal cancer increase with age, and although it is not a strictly menopausal disease, women need to start thinking about screening issues at about the time when they are becoming menopausal. We should be performing annual rectal examinations on our patients in their forties.

If a woman has a direct family history of colorectal cancer, most gastro-enterologists recommend first screening at around 10 years earlier than the age of the youngest relative who was diagnosed with the disease, or age 50 years, whichever comes first. Without a family history, most gastro-enterologists recommend first screening at the age of 50 years. Other risk factors for colon cancer include chronic constipation, eating a highly meat-based diet, obesity, or a history of breast, endometrial or ovarian cancer.

The next question concerns which screen to use. We tell our patients that we would defer to their gastroenterologist as to which test (colonoscopy or sigmoidoscopy) is preferable. Most gastroenterologists make their recom-mendations on the basis of family history, symptoms and dietary risks. Many patients are afraid of the sigmoidoscopy, which is usually performed without anesthesia, and some women report that it is uncomfortable, stating that they would prefer the more extensive colonoscopy, for which they will be sedated and more comfortable.

The risks of the procedure (primarily bowel perforation) are rare, but are more commonly seen with the more extensive procedure. The other issue of course is that the more extensive procedure is also the more expensive one, and many HMOs will only pay for a sigmoidoscopy without certain known risk factors being present.

The worst part of either procedure is not the actual procedure itself. It is necessary to have a totally clean bowel for either screening option, and the clean-out procedure tends to be the same for both. Different bowel prepara-tions have been used, but almost all patients feel uncomfortable with the preparation. This is another area in which it is helpful to be a good example to your patients. If you have reached 50 years of age, you need to do your bowel testing. If you are not willing to go for a colonoscopy, you cannot expect your patient to go for one.

Based on the findings at the time of the procedure, the gastroenterologist will usually make recommendations with regard to when to repeat it. Of course, if your patient develops symptoms of bowel disease prior to that point, you will want her to consult with the gastroenterologist sooner.

Bowel health is yet another area in which a healthy lifestyle can help. Most gastroenterologists will recommend a diet that is high in fiber, fruits and vegetables, and low in animal fats (sounds familiar) in order to reduce the risk of colon cancer.

HRT may also have a role in prevention, although no one would recommend it exclusively to protect the bowel. Several studies, including the WHI, have shown a reduction in colorectal cancer of about 30% in long-term HRT users. Although there is no obvious etiology (such as the bone antiresorption properties of estrogen leading to a reduction in osteoporosis), some gastroenterologists feel that estrogen may render bile less 'irritative' to the gut mucosa, and thereby reduce the cancer risk. Nonetheless, estrogen users should still follow the general screening guidelines.

ENDOMETRIAL CANCER

Menopause itself does not increase the risk of endometrial cancer. However, as this is a disease that peaks in the postmenopausal years, it needs to be discussed here, and there are certain perimenopausal management strategies that may reduce the risk of endometrial cancer.

All postmenopausal bleeding needs to be evaluated (as discussed above, you can start with endometrial biopsies, ultrasound examination and hysteroscopy), but you need to rule out endometrial cancer. Certain women carry higher risks than others. As discussed above, risk factors include unopposed estrogen administration, tamoxifen administration, obesity, diabetes, hypertension and nulliparity. The most modifiable factor is of course obesity, and any weight reduction regime will help.

So what types of perimenopausal management strategies can help? In the perimenopause, the ovaries are still making some estrogen. Indeed, at times they make even more than normal. The obese woman is making her own extra ovarian estrogen, by conversion in her fat tissue of androstenedione from her adrenal glands to estrone, which can stimulate her endometrium. However, what is happening in the perimenopause is that the ovaries are ovulating less well and producing less progesterone. Progesterone limits endometrial build-up, and on a cyclical basis will clean out the uterus.

Some practitioners will administer progestins orally every 2 or 3 months, for 10 or 12 days, in order to induce a withdrawal bleed. Many women are concerned that this will prolong the menopause, so you need to explain to them that the progestins will not build up the lining of the uterus. Explain that their

Table 5 Daily dosages of various progestin medications

Medication	Standard dose (mg/day)	Cyclical dose (mg/day)	
Medroxyprogesterone (Provera®)	2.5	5	10
Norethindrone acctate (Aygestin®)[1]	—	2.5	5
Micronized oral natural progesterone (Prometrium®)	100	200	—

[1]Aygestin tablets are easily cut in half to obtain a 2.5 mg dosage
[2]Cyclical treatment means for 12 days every month or two

remaining estrogen has built up the lining, and that the progestin will help to clear it out. We explain progestin therapy as being akin to using a vacuum cleaner every few months. From a theoretical viewpoint, you are limiting endometrial build-up. From a practical viewpoint, this will help to prevent the 'extravaganza' flows that many perimenopausal women will experience, which often lead to significant HRT or emergency dilation and curettage (D&C).

You can use either medroxyprogesterone (Provera), 10 mg daily for 10 to 12 days, norethindrone (manufactured in the USA as Aygestin®), 5 mg daily for 10 to 12 days or natural progesterone (Prometrium), 200 mg for 10 to 12 days (see Table 5). Tell your patient that she should expect her flow within a week of the last tablet. If she starts to bleed before her last tablet, she can stop taking her pills at that point.

One other advantage of this regime is that it will help your patient around vacation times. If your perimenopausal patient has not had a period for, say, 2 or 3 months, and she is headed for the Caribbean next month, she can take a round of progestin, get her menses and be done with them before she goes on her trip. You just need to help her to time things so that she has had her period before her vacation.

When should your patient stop doing progestin withdrawals? As she gets further into the menopause, and her estrogen production is lower, she should stop building up an endometrium. She will then not get a bleed after she takes her progestin – the latter will only withdraw what has been built up. If she goes for one or two withdrawal cycles and fails to bleed, she should do well. If she is extremely obese and continues to bleed, there is reason to continue with this regime.

For your patient who is diagnosed with endometrial carcinoma, much of her therapy will depend on where you are. Some gynecologists have been trained to perform their own surgery for endometrial cancer, while others will automatically refer to a gynecological oncologist. Some will operate on their own patients if they have an early stage of the disease, with a small uterus and a well-differentiated lesion, and are therefore unlikely to require a pelvic lymph-node dissection.

The next question for the menopause clinician is whether a woman who develops endometrial cancer can be allowed to take estrogens after her surgery if she is very symptomatic. There are few data on women taking HRT in these circumstances, and I would recommend that you discuss the issue with the gynecological oncologist who has taken care of the patient. Some will allow it with an early disease, but many will not. Most will recommend using alternative non-hormonal options.

ENDOMETRIAL HYPERPLASIA

The view of endometrial hyperplasia has changed over the past 20 years. Pathologists and gynecologists have become less concerned about simple hyperplasia without atypia. Whereas a few years ago, gynecologists might even have opted to perform a hysterectomy for this condition, currently some will recommend just following this condition, and noting that if you have already performed a D&C, and this is how this condition was diagnosed, you have already cured the patient. Some will even dispute that simple hyperplasia without atypia is a premalignant condition, in that a very small percentage of these women will progress to carcinoma.

If the patient is currently on estrogen, you will need to add more progestin to her regime, or give her less estrogen. If she has been on a cyclical withdrawal regime every 3 months, you will probably want to increase her to monthly withdrawals. If she is on a daily regime you will want to give her more progestin daily. We usually re-biopsy the patient after 3 months, just to make sure that she is free of hyperplasia.

The more problematic patient is the one who has atypia, as it is these women who are at much higher risk of progressing to cancer. Much of your care for these women will depend on your relationship with the patient. If she is very reliable, you can treat her with a substantial dose of progestin, and then repeat her endometrial sampling after 3 months. You also need to emphasize to her that she will continue to require follow-up. If the patient is very unreliable, you may need to consider hysterectomy because of the risk of progression to endometrial carcinoma. Again, you need to consider the basic endometrial cancer risks that are present initially. If the patient is obese, diabetic and hypertensive, she is a high-risk candidate to begin with.

65

Different practitioners have their own favorite progestin regime. Many will use medroxyprogesterone (Provera), 10 mg twice a day for 3 months. Others recommend norethindrone (Aygestin), 5 mg twice daily. Again, the important thing to re-emphasize is that these women need repeat sampling and careful follow-up if you are not proceeding to hysterectomy. Some women will find the significant doses of progestin uncomfortable, and although they originally planned a medical approach, change their minds and opt for surgical intervention. Although a feasible theoretical consideration would be a progestin intrauterine system, such as Mirena, there is not a significant amount of data on this approach.

BREAST CANCER

Breast cancer is similarly not a disease that occurs secondary to menopause, but its incidence certainly does increase with age. We shall discuss breast cancer prevention strategies, diagnosis and the role of HRT.

Breast cancer prevention

There are a few things that the perimenopausal woman can do to reduce her risk of developing breast cancer. Of course, many of the well-known risk factors, such as family history, she cannot change, and at this point she cannot modify her risks by early childbearing. Although the impact of smoking on breast cancer risk is not as profound as for other cancers, it does increase the risk slightly, so this is yet another reason to encourage your patient to try to stop the habit.

Women with high bone density seem to be at higher risk for breast cancer, as do women with increased breast density noted on mammograms. These factors may well be related to higher chronic circulating levels of estrogen.

However, another lifestyle change may help. Over the last few years data have emerged which suggest that regular aerobic exercise, working out more than three times a week, may decrease the incidence of breast cancer (some studies suggest by as much as 30%). There are also data to suggest that obesity contributes to excess risk, which is logical given the fact that fat tissue manufactures estrogen, and therefore the higher the body weight, the more estrogen there will be. Thus it is prudent to recommend to your patient a low-calorie, low-fat diet that is high in fruits and vegetables, and regular exercise, to maximize her breast health.

Breast cancer is one area in which chemoprophylaxis has been shown to be helpful. In the USA, tamoxifen has been recommended to reduce the risk of developing breast cancer. Indeed, the prospective randomized trial of tamoxifen for prophylaxis in the USA was stopped early because of the impressive results that were obtained. The results of similar trials in the UK and Europe were not as overwhelmingly positive, and tamoxifen use for prophylaxis outside the USA is not as popular. Unfortunately, tamoxifen use is associated with a slightly increased risk of thrombophlebitis and uterine cancers. Moreover, some women have hot flashes when on the drug.

There are formulae for calculating one's risk of developing breast cancer. The most popular formula is the so-called Gail model, which takes into account such factors as age, race, age at first childbearing, number of pregnancies, family history (first-degree relatives with breast cancer) and previous breast biopsies which show hyperplasia. If the patient has a number of risk factors, there may be advantages to taking tamoxifen. However, many patients will want to consult with an oncologist before making this decision.

As mentioned above, there is currently an ongoing trial comparing the SERM raloxifene with tamoxifen for breast cancer chemoprophylaxis. This study is called the STAR (Study of Tamoxifen and Raloxifene) trial, and the results will not be known for several years. If the STAR trial shows comparable prophylaxis from raloxifene, use of the latter will increase, as it does not increase the risk of uterine cancers.

Breast cancer detection

The press has done a good job of confusing American women about how best to detect breast cancer. Recent studies have cast doubt on the value of mammography and even self-examination for the diagnosis of breast disease. Since self-examination is free and carries no risk, we still encourage our patients to self-examine their breasts on a monthly basis. As postmenopausally they will not have a period to link it to, we just encourage them to do it on the first day of the month, or on any day that is convenient to remember.

Most of the recent controversy over the value of mammography has focused on women under 50 years of age. Almost all studies have shown that mammography is valuable in women over 50 years, as the mammograms are considerably easier to read. Reassure your patient that although she may read a lot of information on indications for mammography, the data are really controversial for women under 50 years of age, and that for women over 50 years of age it is a good idea and reliable.

If your patient telephones you about a breast mass, ask her to come in so that you can evaluate it. Remember that the number one malpractice suit in the USA is failure to diagnose breast cancer. In the postmenopausal woman, fibrocystic changes tend to become less noticeable, and as the incidence of cancer increases, any suspicious mass requires full evaluation. If the mass is hard and fixed, send the patient immediately to the general surgeon (unless in your area the gynecologists perform breast biopsies; in most areas of the USA, breast surgery is the province of the general surgeons).

If you consider that the mass does not feel suspicious, it is quite reasonable to send the patient for a mammogram (and ultrasound examination if indicated), and then ask her to come back in a month or two for re-evaluation. Obviously if the mammogram is abnormal, the patient will need immediate surgical consultation. However, if imaging studies are normal, re-evaluate the patient in a month or two. If the mass has resolved, then all is well. However, if the mass persists, the patient should then be referred to the general surgeon for consultation, to see whether biopsy is needed. Remember that a negative mammogram does not mean that no malignancy could be present. It is always good to have a working relationship with the surgeons in your town who feel comfortable about dealing with women with breast diseases.

Again, remembering that this is a litigious society, we would encourage you to install in your office some type of recall service if you do not have one in place already. As breast cases are the most litigious of all, we would recommend that if you see a patient who has a mass, you put her details in a tickler file for a call in 2 months. If your patient does not come in for her follow-up examination in 2 months as you had scheduled, ask your secretary to call her up and remind her. If the patient states 'The mass has gone away', then you can document this in the chart, but if she says that the mass is still there, remind her to come in for her examination. She may say something like 'Well, the mammogram was negative', but you must then remind her that mammograms are not 100% diagnostic. We would also put abnormal mammograms that request a follow-up in 6 months in your tickler file for reminder calls as well. It always amazes us how many women need to be reminded to go back for their follow-up mammogram.

OVARIAN CANCER

Ovarian cancer is another disease whose incidence increases with age. There is no particular significance in relation to the menopause. However, as it is a concern of our patients, we must discuss it with them regularly. We need to explain to them that it is because of the increasing risk of ovarian cancer that they require an annual pelvic examination, even if they are not taking HRT. They need to understand that an annual pelvic examination is still the best screening test for ovarian cancer.

The greatest concern we see among our patients is that one of the commonest complaints of peri- and postmenopausal women is abdominal distension. Indeed, at the annual meeting of NAMS a few years ago, there was a plenary session on 'Gas'. Most highly educated women today know that bloating is a common symptom of ovarian cancer, and therefore it is not surprising that many menopausal women express concern that their bloating is secondary to ovarian cancer. They obviously deserve a thorough examination, and if you have any questions, an ultrasound examination is a very reasonable adjunct.

Many patients request a CA-125 test, which is also hugely popular on the Internet. Unfortunately, this test is highly unreliable and has a significant level of both false-positive and false-negative results. The American College of Obstetricians and Gynecologists does not recommend this as a screening test. We explain all of this to any of our patients who request this test, but if they still insist on the test, we will order it (most actually do not want it after we have explained the foibles associated with it). We also explain to them that the new proteomics tests currently being examined offer a much higher specificity and sensitivity, and that these should be available relatively shortly.

Another concern of women is the question of estrogen therapy increasing the risk of ovarian cancer. A couple of papers have shown a possible but very slight increased risk, although the significant majority of the data does not show an increased risk. Therefore the ovarian cancer risk should be only a minimal consideration when making the decision about HRT.

DEMENTIA

Although dementia is rarely a disease of the early postmenopausal years, it unfortunately occurs all too commonly in the later postmenopause, and questions involving the gynecologist arise with regard to any strategies that can help to postpone or prevent this devastating disease. Furthermore, as a higher percentage of Alzheimer's patients are women (women are one and a half to three times more likely to develop Alzheimer's than men), the gynecologist is automatically involved as a woman's care provider.

As we have previously discussed in the section on cognition (see Chapter 2), many women feel that their cognitive powers and memory decline during the perimenopause. Most of the time this is clearly not a case of serious dementia. However, if any of our patients at any time note a significant loss of mental function or memory, we refer them to an appropriate neurologist or neurologically oriented psychiatrist for an assessment with appropriate psychometric testing. The vast majority of the time such a woman will be reassured that she is not developing dementia, and will be told that she may have normal memory loss or that she is manifesting stress in this manner. If it is a very early dementia, she will then be in the appropriate setting for dealing with this. Medications such as tacrine, rivastigmine and donepezil have effects on cholinergic neurotransmission, and may help the symptomatology.

Reports also regularly appear on the preventative effects of NSAIDs on the development of Alzheimer's disease, but these data are not yet definitive.

The main question posed to healthcare providers for menopausal women is whether estrogen helps to prevent Alzheimer's disease. One of the goals of the WHI was to help to answer this question. Current analysis of the WHI data suggests that delayed initiation of HRT (notably postmenopausally) may actually increase the risk of dementia, not decrease it. There have been a few small studies looking at women on HRT, the majority of which do show some preventative advantages in the group on hormones. Unfortunately, many of these studies are skewed, in that the women on HRT tend to be of higher socioeconomic status, go to chess and book clubs more often, and tend to keep their brains more active. All of these factors are known to help in the prevention of dementia. Everytime the newspapers report on a study showing positive results in the prevention of Alzheimer's disease, we receive numerous inquiries about taking estrogen, as in the USA fear of Alzheimer's is about the only thing we have found to be as scary to women as fear of breast cancer. However, we think that we have to be honest with our patients and point out the limitations of the studies. We tell them that this is one more area where they need to stay tuned, as we do not have the final answers yet.

4

Menopause: specific medications

ESTROGEN

We have discussed many approaches to the patient with various menopausal symptomatologies. However, to paraphrase a popular song, 'Nothing does it better' than estrogen. Certainly for hot flashes, sleep disturbances related to hot flashes and discomfort due to atrophic vaginitis, it is estrogen that will relieve your patient's symptoms most promptly and effectively.

Even the staunchest advocate of the WHI will concede that the use of estrogen therapy in the short term (i.e. for a year or two) has minimal hazards, and if you believe them, they will assure you that most menopausal symptoms, such as hot flashes, do resolve within that timeframe. Whether or not they do you must decide, but certainly for acute relief in most women, estrogens will do the trick.

How to decide which estrogen

For the purposes of this discussion we shall assume that we are dealing with a woman who has not had a menstrual period for at least 3 months, and who is in the later perimenopausal time-frame. We have already discussed (in Chapter 2) the early perimenopausal woman with symptoms, who is actually more difficult to manage.

Estrogen basics: patch vs. pill

The first question we ask our patients when they do opt for estrogen is whether they want a pill or a patch. We will discuss the health issues involved, but the first point you need to establish is patient preference, because compliance or continuance is the basic issue in hormone management.

Many patients prefer a pill. They will say 'I am already taking my thyroid pill, so what is the difference in taking one more pill?'. However, some will counter, 'I am already taking so many pills every day, like my vitamins and my calcium, that I would prefer to avoid taking one more pill'. Some will say 'I forget things a lot, so if I could have a patch that needs to be changed once a week, that would be terrific'. Others will say 'I have very sensitive skin, and even when I put a Bandaid on, I break out', and this will encourage you to prescribe a tablet.

From a medical viewpoint, the patch has a theoretical advantage in that it allows constant absorption of estrogen, and to a patient who is extremely sensitive to changes in hormone levels, this is a major advantage. Migraine sufferers are among your most classic candidates, and they tend to do well with a patch. Moreover, the patch does not raise triglyceride levels as occurs with oral estrogen users, so women who are at significant risk for elevated triglycerides, such as diabetics, are very good patch candidates.

From a theoretical viewpoint, the patch, by bypassing the first pass through the liver, should have less of an effect on the production of all liver proteins. Therefore if you have a patient with a vague history of phlebitis (but negative thrombophilia work-up, and you are still comfortable about starting her on estrogens), you may opt for the patch as being theoretically less of an issue (but remember that this *is* theoretical – there is no substantial literature to prove this point).

However, there are advocates who still believe that the pill does increase HDL levels more, which is a good thing, and therefore recommend its use for that reason.

Furthermore, from a physiological viewpoint, transdermal estrogens lead to less of an elevation of sex hormone-binding globulins, and consequently more free estrogen (this is especially relevant in the patient who has refractory hot flashes, but is on oral estrogen).

All of these factors can influence how you guide the patient, but ultimately she must use the product so that it helps her, so the bottom line is her choice. Moreover, when counseling a patient about HRT, you must always remind her that no decision is irrevocable, and if she hates the patch after 1 week, she must call you and you will change the treatment for her.

Estrogen basics: to have a period or not to have a period

Assuming that your patient has a uterus (we shall deal with the symptomatic woman with salpingo-oophorectomy later), you need to discuss with her the issue of progesterone for endometrial protection. What you need to describe to her is that you can give her estrogen every day, and every month or every other month you can give her 12 days of progesterone therapy, and that after she finishes her progesterone she will probably get a period. You can reassure her that after a while her menses are likely to become lighter and lighter (and may disappear altogther – the absence of an expected period will often generate a phone call requiring reassurance).

Some patients really do not want to resume their menses, and would do anything in their power to avoid them. For these patients, a daily combination of estrogen and progesterone therapy will work. This can be in either tablet or patch form, or in one combined pill or two separate ones (depending on the therapy). Most importantly, you must emphasize to the patient that she may have considerable spotting/bleeding during the first 6 months of therapy, and that this will usually resolve without intervention. Some women will say 'I'd much rather have spotting or light bleeding than a period', whereas others will say 'Spotting irregularly is intolerable to me, and I'd rather have a predictable period than irregular spotting'. Again, remember that neither therapy is etched in stone, and you can easily switch the patient from one regime to the other.

You also need to remember that the earlier the patient is in the menopausal process, the more likely she is to bleed on a daily regime. Therefore if your patient who has been on cyclical therapy for a while stops this regime, and then discovers that she wants to go back on to therapy, it is reasonable to discuss with her switching to a daily regime.

It has also been suggested by cardiology-oriented gynecologists that the unfavorable results for cardiac protection generated by the HERS and WHI studies were due to the daily administration of progestins, as opposed to cyclical administration. They believe that cyclical administration of progestins removes less of the benefit of estrogens. These issues are more of a theoretical nature, and there are few hard data to support these assumptions.

Once you have discussed these basic issues with your patient, you can then help her to decide on a particular estrogen.

Obviously, for the patient who is without a uterus, you do not need to prescribe a progestin and be concerned about bleeding issues. With regard to when to start your patient who has a hysterectomy, she will let you know when she is experiencing symptoms. There are some supporters (with data to back them up) of the notion that menopause may occur in general 1 to 2 years earlier than the national average age of 51 years in women who have ovarian conservation at the time of hysterectomy, possibly secondary to

Do you have menopausal symptoms: yes _____ no _____

Are your menopausal symptoms: severe _____ moderate _____ mild _____

What type of symptoms are you experiencing: _____

_____

_____

Do you have family history of:	Yes	No
Osteoporosis	☐	☐
Heart disease	☐	☐
Breast cancer	☐	☐
Other cancers	☐	☐

Have you been diagnosed with any of the following:	Yes	No
Osteoporosis	☐	☐
Blood clots	☐	☐
Heart disease	☐	☐
Breast cancer	☐	☐
Other cancers	☐	☐

Are you under a lot of stress?

Do you exercise regularly?

Do you smoke?

Do you drink alcohol?

Do you consume adequate amounts of calcium and vitamin D?

What medications are you currently taking?

Have you ever taken hormone replacement therapy (HRT)?

Do you take alternatives instead of HRT?

Figure 4 Patient questionnaire: Making the decision to take hormone replacement therapy

Table 6   Estrogen products and their routes of administration

Estrogen product	Administration	Available dosages
Oral dosing (mg)		
Conjugated equine estrogen (Premarin®)	Daily	0.3, 0.625, 0.9 and 1.25
17-Beta estradiol (Estrace®)	Daily	0.5, 1.0, 1.5 and 2.0
Synthetic conjugated estrogen (Cenestin®)	Daily	0.3, 0.625, 0.9 and 1.25
Transdermal (mg/day)		
17-Beta estradiol (Climara®)[1]	Change weekly	0.025, 0.05, 0.075 and 0.1
17-Beta estradiol (Vivelle®)[2]	Change twice weekly	0.025, 0.05, 0.075 and 0.1

[1]Climara patches are also now available in 0.06 mg/day
[2]Vivelle is also available in 0.0375 mg/day

changes in pelvic blood flow at the time of the surgery. There are also some reproductive endocrinologists who believe that women who have hysterectomies are a somehow different group, with different estrogen receptors who will behave differently to women who do not eventually need hysterectomies.

This is one group in which we will measure FSH levels in order to help to assess their stage in the menopause. However, if we have a patient who is highly symptomatic but still has a normal FSH level, we will empirically treat her to evaluate her response.

Oral estrogen replacement therapy

Estrogens alone

There are many different brands of estrogen tablets on the market (for a summary of available estrogen products and their routes of administration, see Table 6). The oldest estrogen available is Premarin, which consists of conjugated equine estrogens. It comes in many doses, ranging from 0.3, 0.45, 0.625, 0.9, 1.25 to 2.5 mg. Because of its wide range of dosages, it is very easy to titrate a patient's level. Although for many years the standard initial dose of Premarin was 0.625 mg, over the last few years and particularly since the publication of the WHI, many women are switching to the 0.3 mg dose.

Premarin is obtained from pregnant mare's urine, and as such is a blend of at least ten different types of estrogens. Many advocates of Premarin believe that it is indeed this blend, including the delta 8,9 dehydroestrone sulfate, which produces the significant relief of menopausal symptoms. Most of the data on the effects of estrogen replacement therapy from many years back were obtained using Premarin, as it was the first estrogen to be produced.

There is a significant group of women who are anxious about taking Premarin and who ask us for 'natural' hormones instead. Despite our assurances that horses are natural but just not plants, these patients really do not want to take Premarin. For people who like the blend of the hormones that make up Premarin, but prefer a plant source, Cenestin® is a conjugated estrogen from plant sources. A new conjugated estrogen called Enjuvia® is scheduled to be launched this year. It will contain an even closer mix of the hormones in Premarin, but will be derived from a plant source. It is slated to have an even wider dosage spectrum at the lower range, including a 0.45 mg dose, which is useful.

There are also several other brands of oral estrogens at the 0.625 mg and 0.3 mg dosages. These include estropipate and esterified estrogens (Menest®). These are also plant-based estrogens, which is relevant for many patients.

The only major drawback to use of any of the conjugated estrogens is that you cannot readily measure a blood estrogen level. In general, we only measure blood estrogen levels if a patient is symptomatic and not responding to a dose of estrogen to which we think she ought to be responding. Most clinical laboratories will only measure a 17-beta-estradiol level, so you may actually have a patient who has a good estrogen level on 1.25 mg of Premarin, but who will have a low serum estradiol level because she is receiving a group of estrogens other than estradiol. She may then pressurize you to increase her estrogen dosage, which may not in fact be the source of her problems.

The major advantage of conjugated estrogens is that they have a relatively long half-life. From a theoretical perspective, 17-beta-estradiol is best given in a twice daily dosage, whereas conjugated estrogens have a longer half-life and a once-a-day dosing strategy works. We find it hard enough to ask a patient to take one pill a day, let alone one twice a day (and then not in conjunction with meals). However, in practice most patients who are taking estradiol do take it once daily and do reasonably well on it.

17-Beta-estradiol is readily available in several dose levels, (namely 0.5 mg, 1 mg, 1.5 mg (for certain brands) and 2 mg tablets). Again the standard starting dose for many years has been 1 mg, but with current trends we are seeing more use of the 0.5 mg dose level. The two major brands on the market are Estrace and Gynediol®.

Estradiol is derived from soy and Mexican yams, and as such is a plant-based product. The major advantage of estradiol, as we have discussed above, is that you can measure a serum level. Occasionally you will find that some patients are either not absorbing or not metabolizing the dose of estradiol that you are giving them, and you will find a very low blood level. These women may benefit from a switch to a transdermal preparation to obviate the absorption issue, or a switch to a conjugated estrogen product.

Again, as we have already mentioned above, it is important to remind your patient who is on a very low dose of estrogen (0.3 mg of conjugated estrogens or 0.5 mg of estradiol) that she needs to be vigilant about ingesting 1000 mg of calcium daily.

A few words on titrating the estrogen dose are relevant here. Women will often ask what are the signs that they are getting too much estrogen, or too little. We tend to start with a small dose and titrate upward until the hot flashes have significantly abated, or until the woman's sleep patterns have returned to normal. Breast discomfort, bloating and other signs of fluid retention are the major signs of too much estrogen. Occasionally, patients will complain that even on a fairly low dose they are experiencing breast discomfort, in which case you really need to balance the dose with their complaints. If breast discomfort is the only complaint, we encourage these patients to decrease their caffeine intake and to add vitamin B_6 (100–200 mg per day), vitamin E (400–600 units per day) and evening primrose oil (two 500 unit capsules per day). This will often relieve their symptoms.

Transdermal estrogens: patches

The first patch to be manufactured in the USA was the Estraderm® patch. It was originally available in dosages of 0.05 mg/day of estradiol (corresponding to approximately 1 mg of oral estradiol) and 0.10 mg/day of estradiol (or approximately 2 mg of oral estradiol daily). The patch consisted of a reservoir of absorbable estradiol, and the reservoir was surrounded by the adhesive. Estraderm patches need to be changed twice weekly. These patches are still available, and some patients find them very helpful indeed.

As patch technology improved, we saw the development of matrix patches – that is, the adhesive that held the patch on the skin contained the estradiol, and a reservoir was no longer needed. These patches are soy-based products, so most patients are reassured by the source. The next advance occurred when Climara patches were manufactured, as these patches only needed to be changed once a week. Although the difference between twice a week and once a week may sound trivial to many practitioners, we find that compliance with a once-a-week patch is significantly higher than that with a twice-weekly application.

Most of the other matrix patches need to be changed twice a week, and are available in various other dosage levels. Vivelle® and Alora® are the two major name brands. Vivelle has produced a very small patch, called the Vivelle-dot. For people who have sensitive skin, this tiny patch (which the company advertises as being 'as small as a postage stamp') can be very helpful. Unfortunately, some insurers will not pay for these patches, and a case must be often made with the insurer.

Patches are available in many dosages (from 0.025 mg/day to 0.1 mg/day) and dosages can be very easily titrated.

Transdermal estrogen gels and lotions are soon expected to enter the market, notably Estrogel® (an estrogen gel) and Estrasorb® (an estrogen lotion), which will provide an alternative to patches and orals.

Vaginal estrogens

Especially since the WHI results were announced, vaginal estrogens have increased in popularity. Although hot flashes do tend to decrease with time, atrophic vaginal symptoms can become more pronounced. The commonest symptom of vaginal atrophy is dyspareunia. This problem also became more pronounced after the introduction of Viagra, as many women whose partners were previously unable to have intercourse could then become sexually active, but vaginal dryness precluded activity.

Fortunately, atrophic problems can be dealt with at any point post-menopausally. Even a woman who has not been sexually active for 20 years can be treated with vaginal estrogen and vaginal comfort can be restored.

Vaginal estrogen creams

Estrogen creams have been the mainstay of vaginal estrogen therapy for many years. The two most widely prescribed products currently available are estradiol cream (Estrace) and conjugated equine estrogen cream (Premarin). They are sold in tubes with a vaginal applicator. The standard dosage is 1–2 g administered vaginally at night. Many women find the 1 g dose sufficient, and any amount exceeding that leaks out the next morning. You should tell the woman not to use the estrogen cream as a lubricant for intercourse, but to use it on a non-intercourse night, basically to enhance the ability of her own vaginal tissue to generate more moisture.

Patients will ask how often to apply the cream. We encourage our patients to experiment – to apply it twice a week and see if they remain comfortable. If they are still uncomfortable, suggest that they try it three times a week. Just as in systemic therapy, you will need to titrate the dose. Some women will still need some additional topical lubricant for intercourse (see Chapter 2). This is fine, and we recommend that they use Astroglide, K-Y Jelly or whatever they need.

Some women are sensitive to the cream itself. If the patient reports irritation from one particular product, we switch to a different brand. It is seldom the estrogen that is bothering them – usually it is the carrier.

The major question that most practitioners ask is 'Do I need to protect against hyperplasia when administering vaginal estrogens?'. There is no correct answer, as there is very little literature on the subject. Vaginal estrogen cream does get absorbed. However, there is no body of literature showing that women develop endometrial hyperplasia from vaginal estrogen cream alone. Some practitioners will advocate giving these women progestins for 12 days every 3 or 4 months, but most do not.

Unfortunately, these creams are expensive, and many of the women for whom we prescribe them are older women on Medicare, whose medications are currently not covered. We encourage patients to shop around because prices can differ widely. Mail-order pharmacies may be the preferable route for some.

Vaginal tablets

Once again, our European counterparts were ahead of us on this product. Vaginal tablets of estradiol (Vagifem) have been available in northern Europe for many years. Although the principle is the same as that of vaginal estrogen cream, the tablets purportedly show less systemic absorption than the creams. However, more importantly, many women prefer the tablets because they are less messy. The manufacturer's directions instruct women to insert the tablets every night for 2 weeks initially. Most women do not need such intense therapy. Again, women should titrate the frequency of application to symptom relief. Most women end up using the tablets two to three times a week. Some women alternate creams with tablets, which is fine. If the woman has atrophic symptoms from her labia, she will need cream to apply to the vulva, as the tablets will not provide local vulvar relief. The product is currently marketed in boxes of 18 tablets, each with an applicator, making usage easy.

Rings

The Estring, a silicone ring impregnated with estradiol which is slowly released into the vagina at a rate of 7.5 µg per day, also comes from northern Europe. The ring is soft – we describe it to patients as being similar to the rim of a very small diaphragm. The patient places it into the vagina herself, much as she would a contraceptive diaphragm. It then can remain in place for 3 months at a time.

Women report that neither they nor their partners are aware of the ring during intercourse, and that it is quite comfortable. For patients who require constant vaginal estrogen the Estring may be ideal. The other advantage besides comfort is that the amount of estrogen which is systemically absorbed from the ring is nil after the first 24 h from insertion, which means that many oncologists will allow their breast cancer patients to use the Estring. This is obviously very important, as many premenopausal women with breast cancer receive chemotherapy which makes them menopausal. These young women can develop very significant atrophic vaginitis, and any method of delivering vaginal estrogen without raising the systemic level is helpful.

Some women are anxious about keeping a 'foreign body' in their vaginas on a regular basis. You can assure them that there have been no reported cases of toxic shock secondary to Estring use. Nonetheless, if they feel anxious about this issue, they will probably prefer not to use the ring. There are also some women who do not feel comfortable inserting and removing the ring themselves. You can either show their partners how to do it for them, or if that is not an option, these patients may come into the office solely for ring changes, which can easily be done by a nurse practitioner.

Recently, a new delivery system was introduced in the USA. Called the FemRing®, it is very different from the EstRing. The FemRing delivers estrogen transvaginally to the blood stream, in levels comparable to the 0.05 mg per day patch. It improves vaginal lubrication. It also delivers a much higher blood level of estrogen than the EstRing. In a woman who still has a uterus, it must be used in combination with progestins to protect the endometrium. Its major advantage is that it only needs to be changed every 3 months.

Tamoxifen: an unusual use

For the unfortunate woman with metastatic breast cancer, at least two research groups have looked at the use of vaginal tamoxifen for relieving atrophic symptoms, and found good results. They recommend one half tablet applied vaginally twice daily. The proposed mechanism of action is of course that as tamoxifen is a SERM, its vaginal activity is estrogenic. At the level of the breast, tamoxifen is an estrogen blocker.

Complementary and alternative options

Many health-food stores sell products which they advertise for vaginal lubrication, and some women state that these work very well for them. There are no significant data showing that these products work, but they do not seem to produce complications.

In Europe, vaginal soy products are available which are fairly popular. Again, the data on effectiveness are limited. However, the risk of adverse effects is small.

PROGESTERONE AND PROGESTINS

One of the authors, Mary Jane Minkin, started practicing gynecology in 1979, just at the end of the estrogen-only era. Life was good then – almost all women liked taking estrogen. However, when data emerged which indicated that estrogen alone increased the risk of endometrial cancer in women with a uterus in place, we reintroduced the issue of bleeding. We also introduced a drug (medroxyprogesterone acetate, or Provera) which approximately 20% of women do not enjoy taking.

When we started to prescribe Provera in the 1970s, the standard dose was 10 mg for 10–14 days each month. The woman would then get a menstrual period. Over the next few years, researchers realized that probably only a dose of 5 mg daily was needed for most estrogen doses (if a patient is taking a very high dose of estrogen for symptom relief, they may still need 10 mg daily).

By the 1990s we began to realize that hyperplasia could probably still be effectively prevented by administering the progestin every other month. And with the advent of very-low-dose estrogen (0.3 mg of conjugated estrogens or 0.5 mg of estradiol) we realized that with the substantially lowered endometrial stimulation associated with these lower doses, one could probably get by with progestin withdrawal every third or even fourth month.

However, many women really did not like getting a period at all, and this led to the introduction in the 1980s of the practice of administering a low dose of Provera (2.5 mg) on a daily basis. The major drawback of daily dosing, as mentioned above, is that many women get significant unpredictable bleeding on these regimes. This needs to be mentioned to your patient before you prescribe this regime for her. A major question that arises because of the bleeding is when one should biopsy the patient who has bleeding on a daily regime. There are about as many answers to this question as there are menopausologists in this country. We do not biopsy our patients routinely before starting therapy, unless there has been an indication to do so, namely abnormal bleeding. If there is a little breakthrough bleeding in the first month on a daily progestin regime, we do not biopsy them. If it persists through a second month, we will often evaluate their endometrium in some way (usually either biopsy or an ultrasound scan). Once we have biopsied the patient, and if bleeding persists for a third month, we do not repeat the biopsy. At this point the patient will often be very demoralized and will want to switch over to a cyclical regime for a while. The good news is that some of the newer daily progestin regimes have lower breakthrough bleeding rates, which does make life easier.

Wyeth-Ayerst was again the first company in the USA to combine estrogens and progestins into one pill, namely the cyclical Premphase® and the daily Prempro. Premphase consists of 0.625 mg of conjugated equine estrogen taken alone daily for 14 days, followed by a combined pill consisting of 0.625 mg of estrogen plus 5 mg of Provera for the next 14 days. Prempro was initially only available in two dosage levels, namely 0.625 mg of estrogen daily plus 2.5 mg or 5 mg of Provera daily. After the WHI results were published, a lower dose of Prempro was introduced, 0.45 mg of Premarin and 1.5 mg of Provera, to be taken daily.

Because of the convenience of taking one pill a day, Prempro became widely popular. However, we need to return to the issue of the woman who does not do well with Provera. Up to 20% of women complain of irritability, breast soreness, difficulty concentrating and a wide variety of other side-effects. For many years, our next mainstay was norethindrone acetate. Norethindrone has the same protective effect on the endometrium, but at least 50% of the women who cannot tolerate Provera do well on norethindrone (Aygestin). For cyclical therapy, we prescribe Aygestin for 12 days. Unfortunately, it is only manufactured as a 5 mg tablet, so we ask our patients to cut the tablet in half to obtain the 2.5 mg dose, which is the dose we usually recommend. Fortunately, there is now a dose of norethindrone available for daily dosing.

However, that still leaves approximately 10% of women who do not tolerate either Provera or Aygestin. Fortunately, we now have commercially available oral natural micronized progesterone. For many years the micronization process was difficult for commercial manufacturers, and one could only obtain this progesterone from private compounding pharmacies. However, the Solvay company introduced this product commercially, and it is now readily available. Some of our patients still prefer the compounded products, but many insurers will not cover these, although they will cover the commercially available product, known as Prometrium, which is available in 100 mg and 200 mg doses. The standard dose for cyclical withdrawal is 200 mg for 12 days.

The main question you must ask the patient for whom you are prescribing Prometrium is whether she is allergic to peanuts. The micronized progesterone in Prometrium is derived from yams, but the product is then dissolved in a peanut oil base. So if your patient is allergic to peanuts, you will still need to deal with a good compounding pharmacy.

You should familiarize yourself with the compounding pharmacies in your area. You should find one that is reliable and which synthesizes standardized doses, meet with the pharmacist, and see what types of products they can help you with. One pharmacy that does well nationally is the Women's International Pharmacy in Madison, WI. They seem to be able to formulate in reliable doses most of the products that our patients need, and they also send medications through the mail.

Although most women will respond well to natural progesterone administered orally, there will still be 1 or 2% who cannot tolerate even oral natural progesterone. What are your other options? You can try vaginal micronized natural progesterone, which is manufactured primarily for infertility patients (who are taking it in the luteal phase and early on in pregnancy to boost uterine progesterone levels). Formerly available as Crinone® gel, it is now also manufactured as Pro-chieve®. For cyclical administration, most practitioners use one applicator of the 4% gel every other night for a total of 12 nights (i.e. six applications). This is an off-label use of the product, but it is widely done. The gel is sometimes bothersome, but most women are willing to put up with it.

There are still a few women who cannot tolerate any systemic absorption of progesterone. The newest addition to our armamentarium comes from Europe, where Mirena (a levonorgestrel-coated intrauterine system) has been available for around a dozen years. Although this is again an off-label usage (as Mirena is intended as a contraceptive), it delivers a protective dose of progestin to the endometrium without producing a significant systemic level. Usage of Mirena for this purpose is increasing in the USA, and a smaller version of the device for postmenopausal women is currently being developed.

Table 7   Estrogen and progestin combination products

Combination product	Available dosages
Oral	
Prempro™	0.45 mg Premarin/1.5 mg Provera; 0.625 mg Premarin/2.5 mg Provera; 0.625 mg Premarin/5 mg Provera
FemHRT®	5 µg ethinyl estradiol/1 mg norethindrone acetate
Activella®	1 mg 17-beta estradiol/0.5 mg norethindrone acetate
Ortho PreFest®	1 mg 17-beta estradiol/0.09 mg norgestimate
Transdermal	
Combipatch®	0.05 mg/day estradiol/0.14 mg/day norethindrone acetate; 0.05 mg estradiol/0.25 mg/day norethindrone acetate

For women who are intolerant of all versions of progesterone and cannot tolerate Mirena (e.g. a nullipara with a stenotic cervix), we administer estrogen alone. These women obviously need to agree to close management, and to report any untoward bleeding. They require biopsies if they bleed, and most practitioners will either biopsy them or at least perform an ultrasound examination on them once a year, followed by further evaluation for any thickened endometrial stripe. Unfortunately, the development of hyperplasia is not uncommon (remember that most trials of estrogen alone report an incidence of up to 20% annually for the development of hyperplasia). You will then be in a dilemma. These women will not take progesterone. You can try tapering them off their estrogen, but many are intolerant of lack of estrogen. Alternatively, you can conservatively follow them with their hyperplasia, but most practitioners feel uncomfortable doing this. In these cases you may end up performing a hysterectomy.

To return to the other combinations that are available for daily dosing, several years ago new estrogen/progestin combinations became available in the USA. There are currently three other combination pills available, and one combination patch (see Table 7). The three available oral combinations are FemHRT® (5 µg of ethinyl estradiol plus 1 mg of norethindrone daily), Activella® (1 mg of 17-beta-estradiol and 0.5 mg of norethindrone daily) and Ortho PreFest® (1 mg daily of estradiol, with a 3-days-on, 3-days-off regime of norgestimate, the same progestin that is available in Ortho's Tri-cyclen oral contraceptive).

There are several theoretical issues that have been touted with regard to the addition of norethindrone as opposed to medroxyprogesterone (as well as the fact that fewer women are intolerant to norethindrone compared with

Provera). Norethindrone may have more bone-protective effects and less adverse lipid effects than medroxyprogesterone. However, from a practical viewpoint, the greatest benefit that clinicians see is a significant decrease in breakthrough bleeding. Several head-to-head comparisons have confirmed most clinicians' beliefs that less breakthrough bleeding is seen on daily norethindrone. Most clinicians do not report a significant difference between breakthrough bleeding on FemHRT and that on Activella.

Although Ortho PreFest was greeted with considerable enthusiasm from a theoretical perspective when it first appeared on the market, given that it was associated with less progestin administration, and that the norgestimate seemed to be a well-tolerated progestin (on the basis of wide experience in oral contraceptive use), its level of clinical acceptance was low because of the high association with breakthrough bleeding (higher than that seen with Prempro). Although some women did well on Ortho PreFest, most patients with persistent breakthrough bleeding abandoned the product because of the bleeding.

For women who prefer the patch modality, the only currently available combination patch is the Combipatch®, which is a combination of estradiol and norethindrone. The Combipatch is available in two dosage levels, delivering a combination of 50 µg of estradiol and either 140 or 250 µg of norethindrone daily. Unfortunately, the Combipatch is only available in one estrogen dose, so you cannot titrate estrogen levels. If you want to add estrogen in a patch form, you need to add either a Climara or a Vivelle patch in whatever dosage level you need. Combipatches need to be changed twice weekly.

There are several new products in phase III trials. A new patch is slated to be introduced which will be a combination of estradiol and levonorgestrel. It will be available in multiple estrogen dosages, making it easier to titrate doses. A new combination of an oral preparation is also in the pipeline, which will combine estradiol with the new progestin drospirenone, which has become quite popular in the oral contraceptive Yasmin. Its popularity is significantly linked to its diuretic properties (drospirenone is derived from the diuretic spironolactone), and it decreases women's complaints of fluid retention secondary to estrogen therapy.

TESTOSTERONE

Although we have already discussed some aspects of testosterone therapy in the section on Decreased libido on page 30, we would like to describe in detail in this section the use of testosterone. Gynecologists in general feel comfortable with the use of testosterone – we have used topical testosterone cream to treat lichen sclerosis et atrophicus (LS and A) for at least 30 years. Most practitioners report at least a 50% success rate in treating LS and A, which is why this substance has remained part of our armamentarium.

As discussed previously, no one knows the full explanation for libido, and some will dispute whether testosterone plays any role. For caregivers (ourselves included) who would like to try testosterone because they believe that it does play some role, we shall discuss different types of use in the following paragraphs.

Unfortunately, testosterone itself needs to be administered in a transdermal, trans-mucous-membrane or injectable form. If you are administering oral testosterone, you are administering methyltestosterone, which has the potential side-effect of causing liver damage. However, at the doses used for women, this risk is very small. There is no oral methyltestosterone-only product available in a dose acceptable for women. There are male doses, available as 10 mg methyltestosterone (Testred®). Women can break up the tablets into quarters, which is inconvenient, but that way they would obtain 2.5 mg of methyltestosterone, which is the higher end of the range of oral testosterone administration for women.

For women who are also taking estrogen, Estratest is a good product. It consists of esterified estrogens and methyltestosterone. The full-strength pill contains 1.25 mg of estrogen and 2.5 mg of methyltestosterone. The half-strength (HS) dose contains half the amount of both (0.625 mg of estrogen and 1.25 mg of methyltestosterone).

The addition of methyltestosterone to estrogen replacement therapy has several other potential advantages. By decreasing the production of sex hormone-binding globulin, you will increase your effective estrogen level. If you have a patient who experiences persistent hot flashes on estrogen alone this might work, without increasing her estrogen dose. Some studies have shown improvement of cognition with testosterone, while others suggest a generalized improvement in a sense of well-being. One of the authors, Mary Jane Minkin, would be remiss in not attributing her early positive feelings about testosterone to her training by her esteemed mentor, the late Dr John McLain Morris, who would regularly tell her, as early as 30 years ago, to 'Give them a little testosterone, they'll all be OK'.

There are several sexology experts who state that for testosterone to work, the patient must be estrogen replete. However, many patients prefer not to take estrogen, but just take testosterone alone. The options for these women are to use oral methyltestosterone in very small doses, or to use the topical applications. As was mentioned earlier, a commercial product called Androgel (testosterone gel) is available which again is a product for male androgen deficiency. If women use this product, they should apply no more than a quarter of a 2.5 g packet daily, and apply it to the skin of the lower abdomen. You can also ask your compounding pharmacy to make up a testosterone gel in a 1 or 2% form, to be applied daily. Although some experts recommend avoiding genital application, many of our patients have used the gel successfully by applying it to the vulva, noting that it seemed to enhance local responsiveness. They have not developed local masculinizing signs, such as clitoromegaly. These creams should be used on a daily basis – they do not seem to work on an 'as-needed' basis (e.g. using them on Saturday night). Many sexology experts also note that you should encourage your patient to use these products for a 3-month trial, as it may take up to 3 months to see the full response. However, if the testosterone does not work during this 3-month trial, it is unlikely to show improvement thereafter.

A testosterone patch for women is currently in development, and trials have shown an improvement in libido with these patches on an experimental basis. Again, there are patches available in male doses, and some gynecologists recommend that their patients use a daily male patch, but keep it on for 6 h or so (although this does get costly). Hopefully the female patches will be available shortly, and will offer our patients another option.

There are areas of the USA, particularly in the south, where injectable testosterone has been popular for many years. Older practitioners who have used it for years state that their patients really like this method, whereas critics say that it gives too high a peak level immediately after administration. It has been widely used in the past.

The major adverse effects of testosterone are masculinizing effects, namely facial hair growth, acne and a deepening of the voice. You can assure your patient that these effects, if they were to arise, develop very gradually, and she will not wake up one morning looking like Osama Bin Laden. However, with the doses of testosterone that are used for women, these effects are unusual. From a health viewpoint, the major adverse effect would be an adverse lipid profile. Some experts do recommend that you check lipid profiles periodically in women who are on testosterone (but of course you should be checking these periodically in any case). If the patient is on oral methyltestosterone, as we discussed, there is a small potential hepatic effect, and some authors recommend checking liver function tests.

Testosterone will never solve all potential sexual issues for any patient, but we believe that it may prove helpful for some women.

DEHYDROEPIANDROSTERONE (DHEA)

Dehydroepiandrosterone (DHEA) is a relatively newly described hormone. Initial work on this substance was actually done by a scientist who is far better known in our business for another contribution, namely his work on RU 486. This is of course Dr Emile Baulieu.

DHEA has really only been looked at during the last 40 years. Its role in libido is even more disputed than that of testosterone. What has been known for many years is that it is synthesized by the adrenal gland, and that for both men and women levels fall over the course of time, with significant declines potentially starting as early as the thirties. Questions have been raised in the past about the potential adverse effects of administering DHEA, including increasing risks of cardiovascular disease and cancer. Most of this concern has now decreased.

The main question is whether administration of DHEA aids libido. Several studies have suggested that it does. You can easily measure DHEA levels and, if they are low, make a good case for administering the hormone. Some practitioners will empirically try replacement therapy. Fortunately, from a cost point of view, as this is an over-the-counter preparation it is fairly inexpensive. Unfortunately, from a quality-control point of view, this is a debit, because you can never know exactly how much DHEA your patient is taking. Talk with your pharmacists and naturopaths about what brands are available locally for your patients, and which of them are from a reliable source. Standard replacement doses to start with are 25 or 50 mg daily. You can remeasure levels in a few months and then adjust the doses accordingly.

Some patients want to know whether they can use both testosterone and DHEA. If you measure the levels of these hormones and find that both are low, there is no reason not to use both. You can remeasure the levels after replacement, and reassess how your patient is doing pharmacologically and clinically. And of course you may find normal levels of these hormones, and no clinical response at all. Obviously in this situation you will then need to reassess your therapy.

OSTEOPOROSIS MEDICATIONS

Although some of the descriptions of the medications that follow are somewhat redundant to the osteoporosis section, we describe them here for ease of reference. All of the antiresorptives that we shall discuss below will increase bone density, some more significantly than others. However, you must remember that bone density is a surrogate marker, much as a lipid profile can be used as a marker for risk of CAD. With heart disease, your end point is myocardial infarction, whereas with osteoporosis it is fracture. Although the different agents discussed below have slightly different effects on bone density, they all seem to have about the same rate for reduction of fracture.

Another point to remember when interpreting bone-density data and fracture reduction is that the largest risk factor for fracture is previous fracture. Therefore it is crucial to treat women with existing fractures, because they are at very high risk of fracturing again. However, any woman with documented osteoporosis even without an existing fracture is at high risk for a primary fracture, and requires therapy. The reason for including these medications here is that gynecologists and other women's healthcare providers are most likely to encounter women at risk. The therapy is reasonably straightforward. However, if you are not comfortable prescribing these medications, you should refer your patient to either a rheumatologist or an endocrinologist.

RALOXIFENE

Raloxifene (Evista) is a selective estrogen receptor modulator (SERM). It is currently the only SERM used both to treat and to prevent osteoporosis. It was first introduced to prevent osteoporosis, and after the results of the large MORE study were reported, it was approved for osteoporosis therapy. The same dose, 60 mg daily, is used for both therapy and prevention.

Studies on raloxifene have centered around vertebral fractures, and it has been shown that you can reduce the vertebral fracture risk by about half. The studies conducted to date have not been powered to show hip fracture reduction. Remember that hip fractures tend to occur in significantly older women, and that the average age in the raloxifene osteoporosis studies is 67 years. However, there is an improvement in bone density in the hips of these women.

Raloxifene is given as a once daily dose, with or without food. The major health risk of raloxifene is an increased risk (about two- or three-fold) of thrombophlebitis, almost exactly what is seen with estrogen replacement therapy. And if your patient has been on estrogen replacement therapy and has not had a phlebitic complication, it is less likely that she would develop one on raloxifene.

89

The most notable side-effects are seen in a few people who develop leg cramps on medication, which is not related to thrombophlebitis. Some women will develop hot flashes on raloxifene treatment. The likelihood of developing hot flashes is greater in younger women. As was mentioned previously, when transitioning a patient who has been on estrogen for many years, we like to wean the patient gradually from her estrogen, and then wait at least 1 month (and ideally 3 months, based on current data on the likelihood of developing hot flashes from estrogen withdrawal). If you initiate therapy immediately after stopping the estrogen, the patient is much more likely to be experiencing hot flashes secondary to estrogen withdrawal rather than from the raloxifene. The flashes will usually resolve with time, but if annoying flashes persist, you may need either to stop the medication or to try some of the alternative therapies for hot flashes discussed above.

The major advantages of raloxifene for osteoporosis are the other potential health benefits of the drug. As discussed above, in the osteoporosis studies, women on raloxifene have been shown to have a reduced incidence of breast cancer. This is currently under investigation in the STAR trial, which is a head-to-head comparison of the two SERMs in women at high risk of developing breast cancer. If it is shown to be as effective as tamoxifen for breast cancer reduction, raloxifene may become clinically even more popular than tamoxifen, as it is not associated with any uterine stimulation, whereas tamoxifen has been associated with a small risk of uterine cancers.

Raloxifene also has a favorable impact on lipid profiles. It lowers LDL and homocysteine levels, and it does not raise triglyceride or C-reactive protein levels as oral estrogens can. Based on the improvements in lipid profiles, a prospective trial, RUTH, is currently in progress to see whether improvements in these markers correlate with a reduction in cardiovascular disease. The results of the RUTH trial will not be available until 2006.

ALENDRONATE AND RISEDRONATE

Alendronate (Fosamax) and risedronate (Actonel) are both bisphosphonates. Although alendronate use started in the early 1990s, the parent compound of the family, Didronel (etidronate), has been used to treat Paget's disease since the 1970s. Bisphosphonates have also been used for both prevention and therapy of osteoporosis, with excellent results.

Although both alendronate and risedronate cause a more significant rise in BMD, they also produce a reduction in fracture risk of around 50%. Bisphosphonates have shown reductions in hip fractures as well.

The major drawback to the use of bisphosphonates has been their potential to irritate the esophagus. To minimize that risk, your patient needs to take alendronate or risedronate first thing in the morning with a glass of water, and then remain upright for the next half hour (i.e. she cannot lie down). She can then eat her breakfast. Even with careful adherence to the regime, she may still have exacerbation of gastroesophageal reflux disease-type symptoms. This problem is the main one that necessitates stopping the drug.

When these drugs had to be given on a daily basis, this procedure for administration was quite cumbersome. However, later studies showed that once-a-week dosing is as effective as daily dosing, so taking a bisphosphonate has become much less problematic. The weekly therapeutic dose of alendronate is 70 mg once a week, and for prophylaxis a 35 mg dose is available. Risedronate is marketed as a 35 mg once-weekly tablet. Of course, if your patient prefers daily dosing, or tolerates it better, once a day is fine, and the medications for this regime are still available. The doses for daily alendronate are 10 mg for therapy and 5 mg for prophylaxis. For risedronate, the dose is 5 mg daily.

Two questions arises regularly. If your patient does not have a significant rise in her BMD on estrogen or raloxifene alone, or on a bisphosphonate, can you combine these therapies? And will a combination increase her BMD even more? The answer to both questions is yes. However, although combining a bisphosphonate with raloxifene or estrogen will increase the BMD more, there are no data showing a further significant improvement in fracture reduction, so you may be treating numbers without treating the patient. Hopefully data on this issue will be forthcoming.

CALCITONIN

Calcitonin has been used for many years to treat osteoporosis. It is not approved as a preventive therapy. Of all the medications that are used to treat osteoporosis, it has the least effect on BMD. However, some data have shown a reduction in fracture risk, leading to its approval for osteoporosis.

Some osteoporosis experts consider that the major advantage of calcitonin is that it can reduce bone pain associated with osteoporosis, so if your patient is suffering from significant pain with their disease, this may well be an appropriate drug for them.

Administration of calcitonin differs slightly from that of most other medications. It is given daily as a nasal spray, so if for some reason your patient is unable to tolerate pills, calcitonin would be an acceptable alternative.

PARATHYROID HORMONE

Parathyroid hormone (Forteo) was released on to the market for the therapy of severe osteoporosis in 2003. This is actually the first drug that rebuilds bone, and as such it is an excellent choice for the patient with severe bone loss. The medication is available in a daily injectable form, and is to be used for an 18-month period. The use of parathyroid hormone is generally followed by continuation of therapy with an antiresorptive drug, as described above.

Parathyroid hormone is a very expensive medication. Because of its route of administration, cost and use in the very osteoporotic patient, most gynecologists will not prescribe this medication. However, rheumatologists and endocrinologists have been eagerly awaiting this new medication for therapy of significant osteoporosis. If you do diagnose a patient with significant fractures or severe osteoporosis, remember that this medication is available and make the appropriate referral.

BLADDER MEDICATIONS

Although urinary incontinence problems can be seen at any age, many women at menopause do present with bladder symptoms. As we discussed above, atrophic vaginitis can contribute to these symptoms, but urge and stress incontinence may well require further therapy.

TOLTERODINE

Tolterodine (Detrol®) was introduced in the 1990s for the treatment of urge incontinence. Although therapy had been available for many years in the form of the anticholinergic drug oxybutinin, the original formulation of the latter had many side-effects, primarily dry mouth and (to a lesser extent) constipation.

Tolterodine had the advantage that it blocked the muscarinic activity of the bladder more restrictively, and did not produce the extensive dry mouth seen with oxybutinin. Originally available in a 2 mg dose designed to be taken twice daily, it was soon available in a long-acting (LA) 4 mg dose to be taken once a day.

There are very few restrictions on the use of tolterodine. The only patients in whom it is contraindicated are those with narrow-angle glaucoma.

Because of the ease of use of this type of drug, we often initiate a trial of tolterodine before performing extensive cystometric studies, if the patient presents with a clinical history consistent with urge incontinence. We often initiate therapy in a patient who has a history suggestive of a mixed pattern as well. If she does not respond, then full cystometric evaluation is in order.

OXYBUTININ

As mentioned above, oxybutinin was for many years the mainstay of urge incontinence therapy, but it had significant side-effects. Several years ago, a new formulation of oxybutinin (Ditropan XL®) was released, which had two major advantages over the older preparation. It was a timed-release drug, so that it only had to be taken once a day, and the newer preparation had minimized the dry mouth side-effect of the medication.

The indications for the use of oxybutinin are similar to those for tolterodine. There are patients for whom one preparation will work better than the other, so if we have a patient with whom we have tried tolterodine without full success, we will switch to oxybutinin and vice versa, and will sometimes see success with the alternate drug.

Both medications are 'as-needed' drugs, so the patient does not have to take the medication on a regular basis.

DULOXETINE

For many years the gospel for therapy of bladder symptomatology has been to treat urge incontinence with medications, and to treat stress incontinence with surgery. At the time of writing this book, a new medication is slated to be released which has some effect on stress incontinence. A new medication called duloxetine will be available. Duloxetine was actually developed as an antidepressant, with mixed SSRI and SNRI activity.

This neurological activity actually comes into play at the urethral sphincter, and helps to provide bladder control. Although it does not benefit all women with stress incontinence, some effect has been reported in up to 50% of the women who were treated with the medication.

Duloxetine shows maximal effect within 1 month. We anticipate that this medication will be tried in women who do not want surgical intervention for their stress incontinence, or who would prefer to avoid it if possible. Furthermore, although it remains to be seen, we would anticipate that if a patient had problems with both depression and stress incontinence, duloxetine could be a very successful treatment.

COMPLEMENTARY AND ALTERNATIVE MEDICATIONS

There are obviously dozens of preparations available for relief of the symptoms of menopausal women. Some experts dispute that any complementary approach has sufficient scientific data to back it up. However, there are several products which have some literature to back their efficacy and reasonable safety.

Soy

As we have discussed above, many patients prefer a 'natural approach' to menopausal symptoms. Soy has been used for many years by many women to relieve symptoms such as hot flashes. Many people point to Japan, which has the highest dietary intake of soy in the world, as the country where women report fewest hot flashes. The effects of soy are most probably exerted through its phytoestrogen activity.

One of the major controversies in this country surrounds the use of soy extracts as opposed to whole-bean products. The claim is that Asian women do not eat extracts – they eat soy. The FDA has also endorsed this approach, noting that soy itself may reduce the risk of heart disease, but there are very few data on isolated soy products such as isoflavones.

However, American women often do not do well when they add soy products (including soy milk) to their diets. For these women, products are available that contain isolated isoflavones from soy. These products include Estroven and Healthy Woman, which are now available in regular pharmacies (you used to have to go to the health-food stores to find isoflavone tablets). There are a few studies documenting the efficacy of these products for relief of hot flashes. Most of these isoflavone supplements contain 45–60 mg of isoflavones, which is considered to be equivalent to the isoflavone intake in many Asian diets.

Cohosh

The plant root officially named *Cimicifuga racemosa* has been used by Native Americans in this country for many years, but its popularity for the treatment of menopausal symptoms arose in Germany, where it has been used for the last half century. Its mechanism of action is unclear. Unlike soy, which is a phytoestrogen, cohosh does not seem to relieve symptoms by estrogenic activity.

There are standardized cohosh products, which are marketed in the USA (among other countries) as Remifemin and Estroven. Standard doses of cohosh are 20 mg twice daily. The European literature suggests that therapy should be used for 6 months, and then the need for continuation should be reassessed. Cohosh and soy can be taken together.

Cohosh is one of the few products which in at least some studies seems to relieve hot flashes, and it has minimal side-effects.

Ginseng, ginkgo and dong quai

We mention these herbs together to note that there is very little literature supporting their use for relief of menopausal symptoms. However, many women may be taking them, and you need to be aware of their use, because they can all be associated with increased risk of bleeding. If you are preparing a patient for surgery, you must obtain her entire medication history and encourage her to stop taking herbal preparations, particularly these medications, at least 1 week prior to surgery.

5

Case studies

A.R. is a 45-year-old G1P1 who presented for her annual examination. Her history is remarkable in that she was a longstanding infertility patient, who conceived with high doses of gonadotropins 8 years ago. For the past year she has had very erratic menses, but when they do occur, after a 3- or 4-month interval, she has moderately heavy flow. She has regular hot flashes, and her sleep is very disrupted with night sweats. She is slim, a non-smoker and in general in otherwise very good health. Although she is nominally at the office for her routine visit, she would like some intervention for these symptoms.

It is not surprising to find women who have experienced ovulatory difficulties presenting with slightly earlier than average perimenopausal symptoms. This may be consistent with the old observation that the later the menarche, the earlier the menopause (due to less 'robust' ovaries). A.R. is an ideal candidate for oral contraceptives. She is not fully menopausal, but she is quite symptomatic. The oral contraceptives also have the advantage of offering her some reduction in ovarian cancer risk. She is currently at somewhat increased risk given that she had only one child, as a result of significant FSH therapy.

With regard to which pill to choose, really any 20–35 μg pill would be reasonable. In these circumstances, we gave her Mircette, a 20 μg pill which is packaged with five estradiol tablets in lieu of the last five placebo pills, which reduces menopausal symptoms during the withdrawal week.

The next question is how long to maintain this patient on the pill. We would keep her on it for anywhere between 6 and 12 months, and then stop the pill and reassess her condition. If she were then fully menopausal, we would reassess her symptoms for consideration of HRT. If she were not, we could reinstitute oral contraceptive therapy.

N.N. is a 50-year-old G3P3 who has intermittently experienced menorrhagia in the past. However, she had been doing well until her menses became more erratic. She now goes for about 2 months without a period, and then floods. We checked her hematocrit, which is now 31%. She weighs 200 pounds, is a non-smoker and has no other menopausal symptoms. Her husband has had a vasectomy.

N.N. is a good candidate for periodic progestin withdrawal. Although you could offer her oral contraceptives, she most likely would do well with just monthly administration of progestins (medroxyprogesterone, 10 mg for 7–10 days, or norethindrone, 5 mg for 7–10 days) to produce a withdrawal bleed. However, before administering progestins, we would perform an endometrial biopsy in the office to rule out any endometrial pathology. You need to reassure such patients that progestins will not prolong their menopause, and we explain that we think of them as being like a vacuum cleaner, just clearing out tissue that has already built up. You should explain to them that as they get further into the menopause, their withdrawal bleeds will lessen and then cease, as their estrogen levels decline. This method is nothing more than a variant of Dr Gambrell's progestin challenge test, which he administered every 3 months until women ceased to get withdrawal bleeds.

Of course, you should always counsel overweight patients to adhere to a low-fat and low-cholesterol diet, and to exercise as much as possible. This patient's menorrhagia would also respond to weight loss.

J.L. is a 44-year-old woman who presents with night sweats and hot flashes. She is a G1P1, and has always been slender. Her mother underwent an early menopause, so she is not surprised that she is having night sweats already. Her menses have become more erratic, and she is getting relatively light periods every 2–3 months. After discussion of the various options, J.L. decides to try oral contraceptives. After 1 month she does get a withdrawal bleed, but she states that she feels no better on the therapy. Her sweats are now worse than they were. She stops the oral contraceptives and continues to feel poorly. At this point, you draw some blood tests and find that her FSH is 10 mIU/ml and her estradiol is 50 pg/ml. However, you also draw a set of thyroid function tests and find that her TSH level is undetectable and her free T_4 level is markedly elevated.

J.L. is an example of a woman with presumed early menopausal symptoms who logically presents to her gynecologist, but turns out to have non-gynecological disease. When a woman fails to respond to the estrogen therapy you have instituted, you need to exclude other medical disease states. Thyroid disease is relatively common in women, and occasionally we see the hyperthyroid presentation. Currently J.L. is well controlled, although her eyes now show the changes of Graves' disease, which she did not have on initial presentation.

N.T. is a 54-year-old woman who has been on HRT for 3 years. Therapy was started because she was significantly symptomatic while going through the menopause. She is upset because she has just had an abnormal mammogram which showed an area of asymmetric density. The radiologist requested a follow-up film in 6 months. She also has a family history of osteoporosis, which is one of the reasons why she initiated HRT. You discuss the various options, and she decides to taper off the HRT, and does well. You have sent her for a bone density study, which shows a T score in her hip of –2. She is somewhat anxious about this, given her mother's history. What options might you offer her?

N.T. would seem to us to be the ideal candidate for raloxifene therapy (Evista). Raloxifene has shown a substantial reduction in fracture risk, comparable to bisphosphonate therapy. However, the added advantage here is that raloxifene does reduce breast density in mammography studies, and may offer the woman a reduction in her risk of breast cancer. Thus you could offer her several advantages with one therapeutic option.

Follow-up: N.T. does well with her raloxifene therapy. However, at her next year's visit she complains of vaginal dryness. What can you offer her?

N.T. would be an excellent candidate for vaginal estrogens in either cream, tablet or ring formulation, depending on her preference. There is no contraindication to the use of vaginal estrogens with raloxifene. Initially you would ask her to use the medications every night or every other night for a 2-week period, and then you would have her titrate her usage, depending on symptom relief.

We present the following case as an example of what we used to do, compared with what we might do now.

D.R. was a 52-year-old newly menopausal woman. Although she did not have a lot of formal education, she was a very intelligent woman who read extensively. She presented us with the following history about 8 years ago. She had already had a coronary bypass procedure performed at the age of 48 years. Her two brothers had died of CAD at very young ages. Her mother also died of CAD at the age of 55 years, and in addition her mother had had a mastectomy for breast cancer at the age of 47 years. Her 50-year-old sister had also just had a mastectomy. Her question to us was which was more important – her history of CAD or her family's history of breast cancer? We obviously discussed this at length, and she decided to initiate HRT. She started taking estradiol, 1 mg daily, and oral natural progesterone, 100 mg daily. When the HERS study was published, she had already been on estrogen for about 4 years, so we opted to keep her on the estrogen. We revisited the issue recently. She had done very well from both a cardiac and breast health point of view. When discussing the pros and cons, D.R. opted to continue to take HRT, saying 'No one in my family has ever reached 60 before – I don't want to rock the boat'.

Of course, if such a patient were to present today, we would not encourage her to take HRT for cardiac prophylaxis. It will be interesting to see the results of the RUTH and STAR trials. If these do show cardiac and breast benefits, a patient such as D.R. would be a good candidate for raloxifene treatment.

S.M. is a 53-year-old G2P2 who is coming in for her annual visit. She comments that she has not had a period since her last yearly visit. She is experiencing some hot flashes, but friends of hers have suggested that she should try soy therapy and black cohosh, and she has done well with these for symptom control. Her history is remarkable in that she was a smoker for 15 years. However, she stopped smoking when she developed asthma. She is intermittently on doses of prednisone. She also had a history of thrombophlebitis many years ago during her second pregnancy. She wants to know where she should go from here.

S.M. clearly needs some advice. Our major concern about someone with this history would be her osteoporosis risk. She has a history of smoking, and she is intermittently taking steroids, both of which are predisposing factors for osteoporosis. She would be a good candidate for a bone-density test to establish her baseline. Even if she has no bone loss now, she requires counseling about the need to take 1500 mg of calcium and 400 units of vitamin D a day, and to follow a good weight-bearing exercise program.

If S.M. has osteoporosis already, all would agree on the need for intervention. If she has osteopenia, many experts would counsel in favor of intervention, and some would recommend regular bone densitometry. If you did want to start medication, S.M. would be an ideal candidate for bisphosphonate treatment. You would want to avoid estrogen and raloxifene because of her phlebitis history, and there is no role for calcitonin for prophylaxis. She should do well with weekly alendronate or risedronate.

Index